The Handbook for
EVIDENCE-BASED
PRACTICE in
COMMUNICATION
DISORDERS

The Handbook for
EVIDENCE-BASED
PRACTICE in
COMMUNICATION
DISORDERS

by

CHRISTINE A. DOLLAGHAN, PH.D., CCC-SLP
University of Texas at Dallas

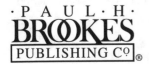
·P·A·U·L·H·
BROOKES
PUBLISHING CO.®

Baltimore • London • Sydney

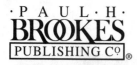

Paul H. Brookes Publishing Co.
Post Office Box 10624
Baltimore, Maryland 21285-0624

www.brookespublishing.com

Typeset by Spearhead Global, Inc., Bear, Delaware.
Manufactured in the United States of America by
Versa Press, Inc., East Peoria, Illinois.

The case studies in the book represent hypothetical situations, and any resemblance to real people is unintended.

Fifth printing, September 2015.

Library of Congress Cataloging-in-Publication Data

Dollaghan, Christine A.
   The handbook for evidence-based practice in communication disorders /
by Christine A. Dollaghan.
      p. ;   cm.
   Includes bibliographical references and index.
   ISBN 978-1-55766-870-7 (alk. paper)
   1. Communicative disorders—Treatment.   2. Evidence-based medicine.
I. Title.
   [DNLM: 1. Communication Disorders.   2. Evidence-Based Medicine. WL
340.2 D665h 2007]
   RC423.D65 2007
   616.85′5—dc22   2007017769

British Library Cataloguing in Publication data are available from the British
Library.

Contents

About the Author. vii

Preface ix

Acknowledgments xi

1   Introduction to Evidence-Based Practice 1

2   Asking Questions About Evidence 9

3   Finding External Evidence. 17

4   Validity of Evidence: An Overview. 27

5   Importance of Evidence: An Overview. 47

6   Appraising Treatment Evidence 63

7   Appraising Diagnostic Evidence 81

8   Appraising Systematic Reviews and Meta-Analyses. 105

9   Appraising Patient/Practice Evidence 113

10   Appraising Evidence on Patient Preferences 123

11   A Prognosis for E³BP in Communication Disorders. 133

References 139

Appendix A   CATE: Critical Appraisal of Treatment
             Evidence 153

Appendix B   CADE: Critical Appraisal of Diagnostic
             Evidence 155

Appendix C   CASM: Critical Appraisal of Systematic
             Review or Meta-Analysis 157

Appendix D   CAPE: Checklist for Appraising Patient/
             Practice Evidence. 159

Appendix E   CAPP: Checklist for Appraising Evidence
             on Patient Preferences 161

Index 163

About the Author

Christine A. Dollaghan, Ph.D., CCC-SLP, Professor, University of Texas at Dallas, School of Behavioral and Brain Sciences, Callier Center on Communication Disorders, 1966 Inwood Road, Dallas, Texas 75235

In 2006, Dr. Christine Dollaghan joined the faculty of the University of Texas at Dallas, where she conducts research and teaches in the areas of pediatric communication disorders and evidence-based practice. Dr. Dollaghan began presenting workshops and courses on evidence-based practice to speech-language pathologists and audiologists in 2002 and has taught on this topic nationally and internationally. Her broad research interests concern the conditions and processes that enable children to learn the language that surrounds them—both when their learning proceeds seamlessly and when it breaks down. Her recent research has addressed questions about the validity of diagnostic categories and diagnostic measures, the impact of biological and sociodemographic variables on children's language development, and the predictors of speech and language outcomes in children developing typically and in children with severe traumatic brain injury. Dr. Dollaghan is a Fellow of the American Speech-Language-Hearing Association (ASHA), was an associate editor of the *Journal of Speech, Language, and Hearing Research,* and served for 5 years as a member of the Behavioral and Biobehavioral Subcommittee of the National Institutes of Health. She chaired ASHA's Research and Scientific Affairs Committee from 2001 to 2004 and in 2007 will have completed a 3-year term as chair of ASHA's Advisory Committee on Evidence-Based Practice.

Preface

When I first started reading about evidence-based medicine in 1999, I was amazed and energized. I was amazed that I knew so little about these ideas, and energized by their potential to move us closer to answering fundamental questions about communication disorders that have been debated but not resolved for many years. As I've gone on to learn and teach about the evidence-based orientation, I've been delighted to discover how many other clinicians, students, and faculty in speech-language pathology and audiology also find themselves intrigued by this way of thinking. However, there was no single source of basic information about evidence-based practice that I could recommend to those interested in pursuing these ideas with reference to communication disorders. This handbook synthesizes the information that I have found most helpful into a framework that I hope will inform as well as energize readers at all levels.

The handbook does not report the "current best evidence" in communication disorders; such evidence is destined to change far too rapidly for this to be a reasonable goal for a text. Instead, it provides a foundation for thinking about the quality and strength of evidence that is relevant to any and all questions about clinical decision making. Readers of the book should be able to confidently conduct their own explorations of the evidence in their specific areas of interest. The handbook offers something like a simple, portable map of the evidence landscape as we understand it currently—a starting point that will need to be annotated and revised as we work together to develop a clearer view of the terrain.

Acknowledgments

Barbara Bain, Lesley Olswang, and Tom Campbell contributed directly to my initial interest in the quality of clinical evidence; I thank them for many thought-provoking discussions over the years. It has also been my good fortune to work with Jack L. Paradise, Janine Janosky, and Howard Rockette; I hope that a few glimmers of their reflected wisdom can be found in this book. Tony Delitto has my undying gratitude for introducing me to the work of David L. Sackett, which led me in turn to the literature on evidence-based medicine. Finally, my colleagues and friends on several committees of the American Speech-Language-Hearing Association provided extremely helpful insights, criticisms, and support. Randy Robey, Brenda Lonsbury-Martin, Travis Threats, Ron Gillam, John Grose, Ray Kent, Brian Shulman, Mary Pat Moeller, Celia Hooper, Barbara Ehren, Tom Helfer, Julie Masterson, Tracy Schooling, Tobi Frymark, Marc Fey, and Rob Mullen deserve my particular thanks, along with my apologies for any of their ideas that I've misrepresented or failed to acknowledge adequately.

At Paul H. Brookes Publishing Co., Elaine Niefeld talked me into this project, and Astrid Zuckerman, Johanna Cantler, and Trish Byrnes talked me through it. I owe them all an enormous debt of gratitude.

Finally, Tom Campbell, Annicka Campbell-Dollaghan, and Kelsey Campbell-Dollaghan provided me with an endless supply of encouragement and music. I thank them most of all.

For my parents, Art and Nancy Dollaghan

1

Introduction to Evidence-Based Practice

If it is a miracle, any sort of evidence will answer, but if it is a fact, proof is necessary.

—Mark Twain, American writer

EVIDENCE-BASED PRACTICE: AN EXPANDED DEFINITION

It sometimes seems as though evidence-based practice (EBP) is taking over the world. EBP is a key topic of discussion (and controversy) in fields as diverse as clinical laboratory science (e.g., McQueen, 2001), nursing (e.g., Rutledge, 2005), physical medicine and rehabilitation (e.g., Cicerone, 2005), occupational therapy (e.g., Tse, Lloyd, Penman, King, & Bassett, 2004), psychology (e.g., Wampold, Lichtenberg, & Waehler, 2005), psychiatry (e.g., Hamilton, 2005), and education (e.g., Odom, Brantlinger, Gersten, Horner, Thompson, & Harris, 2005). Sessions on EBP began appearing on the program of the annual convention of the American Speech-Language-Hearing Association (ASHA) in 1999, and the move toward EBP has been endorsed in an ASHA technical report (ASHA, 2004) and position statement (ASHA, 2005a). An evidence-based orientation can even be found in a book about the success that resulted for a baseball team when prospective players were evaluated with objective performance measures in addition to the subjective impressions of baseball scouts (Lewis, 2003).

Its rapid spread notwithstanding, EBP has generated negative as well as positive reactions. Most criticisms can be traced to several problems with the way that the phrase has come to be understood. One problem is that the EBP "movement" seems to imply that until EBP came along, practitioners were basing their clinical decisions on something other than evidence, which is simply not true. In addition, most people seem to think that EBP involves only

1

research evidence, which also is not true. Sackett, Rosenberg, Gray, Haynes, and Richardson (1996) originally defined *evidence-based medicine* as "… the conscientious, explicit, and judicious use of current best evidence in making decisions about the care of individual patients … [by] integrating individual clinical expertise with the best available external clinical evidence from systematic research" (p. 71). Both research evidence and clinical expertise were a part of this original definition, and a third component (the patient's perspective) was added to the subsequent definition of EBP as ". . . the integration of best research evidence with clinical expertise and patient values" (Sackett, Straus, Richardson, Rosenberg, & Haynes, 2000, p. 1). Despite the inclusion of clinical expertise and patient values in definitions of EBP, it is clear that the emphasis on scientific evidence has overshadowed the other two components.

As a way of bringing all three components into focus, I'd like to suggest that we think of EBP as requiring not one but three kinds of evidence, and the abbreviation E³BP will be used to help keep all three types of evidence in mind. Accordingly, the definitions discussed previously will be adapted (Sackett et al., 1996, 2000), and in this handbook we will define *E³BP* as the conscientious, explicit, and judicious integration of 1) best available *external* evidence from systematic research, 2) best available evidence *internal* to clinical practice, and 3) best available evidence concerning the preferences of a fully informed patient.

This definition will allow us to circumvent several criticisms and confusions that have bedeviled the previous concept of evidence-based practice and its progenitor, evidence-based medicine (e.g., Cohen, Stavri, & Hersch, 2004; Rees, 2000). For one thing, the definition of E³BP clearly distinguishes between external and internal sources of strong evidence and highlights the importance of both for clinical decision making. Evidence internal to clinical practice with a particular patient is an important complement to external evidence from systematic research because although high-quality external evidence can reveal valuable information about average patterns of performance across groups of patients, its applicability to an individual patient is unknown (Bohart, 2005). Conversely, high-quality internal evidence from clinical practice with an individual patient is surely relevant to making decisions about that patient (Guyatt et al., 2000), although its applicability to other patients or groups of patients is likewise unknown.

Those who work in behavioral sciences, and especially in communication sciences and disorders, have an advantage when it comes to obtaining strong internal evidence because of experience with well-developed single-subject methodologies (e.g., Horner, Carr, Halle, McGee, Odom, & Wolery, 2005) for measuring change in individual patients. Although the need for such methods is clear, Sackett et al. (2000) acknowledged that the use of such methods in medicine is in its infancy. The expanded definition emphasizes that strong evidence internal to clinical practice can and must be incorporated to make E³BP a reality in communication disorders.

Finally, E³BP also requires strong evidence about our patients' beliefs, preferences, hopes, and fears (e.g., McMurtry & Bultz, 2005) concerning the clinical options that face them. To paraphrase Sullivan (2003, p. 1595), "facts known only by practitioners need to be supplemented by values known only by patients." Incorporating this third type of evidence requires that we develop a shared understanding of our clients' perspectives, as well as ensuring that clients comprehend their clinical alternatives so that they can express meaningful preferences.

You may have noticed that the expanded definition of E³BP does not refer specifically to clinical expertise, which was a key component of the original definitions by Sackett et al. (1996, 2000). That is because in my view clinical expertise is not a separate piece of the E³BP puzzle but rather the glue by which the best available evidence of all three kinds is integrated in providing optimal clinical care.

PRECONDITIONS TO E³BP

According to this expanded definition, successful E³BP has three preconditions:

1. Uncertainty about whether a clinical action is optimal for a client

2. Professional integrity (comprising honesty, respectfulness, awareness of one's biases, and openness to the need to change one's mind)

3. Application of four principles that underpin clinical ethical reasoning: beneficence (maximizing benefit), nonmaleficence (minimizing harm), autonomy (self-determination), and justice (fairness)

Thus, E³BP requires honest doubt about a clinical issue, awareness of one's own biases, a respect for other positions, a willingness to let strong evidence alter what is already known, and constant mindfulness of ethical responsibilities to patients (e.g., Kaldjian, Weir, & Duffy, 2005; Miller, Rosenstein, & DeRenzo, 1998).

The crucial role of uncertainty in E³BP is worth emphasizing. Seeking evidence not in an effort to reduce honest uncertainty but rather in an effort to prove what one already believes is contrary to the fundamental thrust of E³BP. It is also likely to be a waste of time, because any contradictory evidence will be ignored or discounted in favor of evidence that supports one's point of view.

Awareness of the powerful and distorting effects of subjective bias has been a major impetus for the evidence-based orientation. All people have biases or preconceived notions that frame, organize, and often simplify their perception of the world. Francis Bacon was one of the first to address the ways in which biases can weaken the ability to seek, recognize, and acknowledge strong evidence.

> The human understanding, once it has adopted opinions, either because they were already accepted and believed, or because it likes them, draws everything else to support and agree with them. And though it may meet a greater number and weight of contrary instances, it will, with great and harmful prejudice, ignore or condemn or exclude them by introducing some distinction, in order that the authority of those earlier assumptions may remain intact and unharmed. (1620, cited in Meehl, 1997a, p. 94)

In short, our strong preference for what we already believe to be true makes us poor judges of whether it actually is true.

How important is it to test the validity of subjective beliefs? That depends at least partly on their consequences. Testing the validity of a personal belief (say, in the existence of extraterrestrials) is not important if that belief has no impact on other people. But when a belief has the potential to harm other people, testing its validity is imperative. Meehl (1997a) provided an example in his description of the *Malleus Malleficarum*, a book published in 1487 that addressed an important diagnostic problem at the time: how to identify witches. Meehl noted that its authors were respected experts who grounded their detailed list of diagnostic indicators firmly in what was known at that time—that witches existed, that they were dangerous, and that they needed to be identified in order to protect innocent people. Despite the authors' good intentions, of course, their work actually led to enormous harm for many innocent people who were diagnosed as witches and then treated by drowning, burning at the stake, and so forth. Only when these widely accepted, expert views about witches were tested using more objective criteria did belief in them gradually wane.

As many have noted (e.g., Barrett-Connor, 2002; Meehl, 1997a; Sackett, Haynes, Guyatt, & Tugwell, 1991), it is not difficult to find more recent examples of clinical recommendations that, although based on the beliefs and good intentions of experts, turned out to be ineffective or even harmful when subjected to rigorous scientific testing. The newspaper this week probably contained at least one such report. Growing awareness of the limitations of subjective beliefs, even from experts, as a basis for decisions about patients' lives explains why external evidence from scientific research is one of the three cornerstones of EBP. Although complete objectivity may be an unrealistic goal (e.g., Hegelund, 2005), the idea that evidence should be as free as possible from the distorting effects of an observer's subjective bias(es) or expectations is one of the most important contributions of the evidence-based perspective.

The significance of avoiding subjective biases, especially when they might result in harm, also is related to four principles of clinical ethical reasoning (e.g., Kaldjian, Weir, & Duffy, 2005). The principle of *beneficence* obligates us to practice in a manner that is maximally beneficial to our patients. The principle of *nonmaleficence* obligates us to avoid harming our patients. The principle of *autonomy* (a relatively recent addition in the literature on medical ethics) obliges us to respect the right of patients to have the power to determine what happens to them based on a full understanding of the risks and benefits of the options that face them. The principle of *justice* obliges us to practice in a fair, nondiscriminatory manner. You might be familiar with these principles in connection with the protection of human subjects in research because balancing potential benefits and harms is a topic of well-publicized discussion when participants are harmed by research. However, these same principles apply to the protection of patients during clinical practice, and they can be particularly helpful in situations in which the best available evidence from external research, from clinical practice, and from a fully informed patient does not converge neatly on the same clinical decision.

ORIGINS AND EVOLUTION OF EVIDENCE-BASED PRACTICE

With the definition and preconditions of E^3BP in mind, it is time for some historical context. How and why did the evidence-based orientation originate? The enormous increase in research literature, in medicine, and in other fields was one major impetus (Sackett et al., 2000). For example, a recent search for information on communication disorders in PubMed, an electronic database, yielded a total of nearly 40,000 citations, and about 8,000 of these were to articles published in the past 5 years. The sheer number of publications presents practitioners with a serious challenge in finding and using the information they need in making decisions about their patients' health. One of the original goals of evidence-based medicine was to assist practitioners in rapidly finding and using the wheat available in the literature and spending a minimum amount of time with the chaff.

The evidence-based framework has also been compelled by the lack of unanimity that is a common feature of the research literature concerning a particular clinical question. Because findings, conclusions, and clinical implications from different studies often vary, clinicians needed a systematic, defensible, and practicable process for deciding which external evidence should carry the most weight in their decision making. This need has resulted in more than 100 systems for rating external evidence (Lohr, 2004). All such evidence-ranking schemes involve a set of criteria for evaluating the quality of evidence so that the best current external evidence can be identified readily, consistently, and transparently.

Rating External Evidence: The Oxford Hierarchy

One of the first, most comprehensive, and most influential systems for rating evidence is the Oxford Centre for Evidence-Based Medicine Levels of Evidence (Phillips et al., 2001; http://www.cebm.net/levels_of_evidence.asp). One of the strengths of the Oxford system is its explicit acknowledgment that no single set of criteria applies to every kind of evidence, and different rating criteria are needed according to whether evidence concerns treatment, prognosis, diagnosis/screening, differential diagnosis, and health care economics.

The working group responsible for the Oxford system characterized it as a work in progress and acknowledged one weakness of the system—its emphasis on the internal validity of external evidence and particularly on research design as the primary basis for assigning evidence to a level. As shown in Table 1.1, for example, evidence concerning therapy that was derived from expert opinion without critical appraisal, or by induction or inference alone, is ranked lowest (Level 5) because of its potential to be affected by subjective bias and other sources of error. At the other end of the hierarchy (Level 1a) is evidence that has been found consistently across multiple studies conducted so as to minimize the potential for results to be contaminated by subjective bias or other sources of error.

Table 1.1. Some of the levels in the Oxford Centre for Evidence-Based Medicine Levels of Evidence for studies of therapy

Level	Description
1a	Systematic review of two or more high-quality randomized controlled clinical trials (RCTs) showing similar direction and magnitude of results
1b	Individual high-quality RCT with results surrounded by a narrow confidence interval
2a	Systematic review of two or more high-quality cohort studies showing similar direction and magnitude of results
2b	Individual high-quality cohort study or low-quality RCT
2c	Outcomes research; ecological studies
3a	Systematic review of case-control studies showing similar direction and magnitude of results
3b	Individual high-quality case-control study
4	Case series or poor quality cohort or case-control studies
5	Expert opinion without explicit critical appraisal, evidence from physiology, bench research, or first principles (i.e., axiomatic)

Source: Phillips et al. (2001).

Although these "quality extremes" are easy to recognize, most empirical evidence falls somewhere in-between, and the characteristics that distinguish among the intermediate levels are not always transparent. Research design (i.e., whether a study is a randomized controlled trial, a cohort study, a case study, and so forth) is the most salient factor that differentiates the levels, but qualifiers such as good quality, poor quality, and well conducted are also used to distinguish among levels in the Oxford system. Many of the additional quality indicators are discussed in the evidence-based medicine literature, but as of this writing they have not been incorporated explicitly into the original Oxford system. Accordingly, many subsequent evidence rating systems have failed to include factors other than research design in their criteria for evaluating evidence. In fact, research design is so heavily emphasized in extant evidence-rating schemes that it is easy to make the mistake of thinking that certain kinds of designs guarantee high-quality evidence. In reality, studies with highly ranked designs can yield invalid or unimportant evidence just as studies with less highly rated designs can provide crucial evidence. It is increasingly clear that "even within randomized controlled trials, quality is an elusive metric" (Berlin & Rennie, 1999, p. 1083) and one that may not be reducible to a single numeric rating (Glasziou, Vandenbroucke, & Chalmers, 2004).

Later in this handbook you will learn how to weigh several dimensions of quality, not just research design, in deciding which external evidence should influence your clinical decision making. For now, two points about evidence-level schemes need to be emphasized. First, assigning evidence to a level requires knowing more than the type of research design employed in the study from which the evidence came. Second, characterizing evidence with a single numerical rating too often encourages an all-or-none mentality in which evidence with a rank lower than the top is completely discounted and evidence from a study at the highest rank is assumed to be definitive. As we will see, neither one of these perspectives is accurate.

This is a good place to clarify another point of confusion about evidence-based practice—that it does not require or depend on clinical practice guidelines (CPGs) that have been defined as "systematically developed statements to assist practitioner and patient decisions about appropriate health care for specific clinical circumstances" (Institute of Medicine, 1990, p. 38). CPGs ideally result from the efforts of a broadly representative and skilled group of individuals who conduct a comprehensive literature search for evidence relevant to answering one or more well-formulated questions about a particular clinical condition, conduct independent critical appraisals of the existing literature using well-specified criteria, summarize the strength of the evidence concerning the benefits and harms of specific courses of clinical action, and synthesize their findings into a set of recommendations reflecting the strength of the scientific evidence for or against the alternative courses of action. Systematic reviews and meta-analyses (which will be discussed later) also review, critique, and synthesize the literature on a topic, but unlike CPGs, they do not reflect the additional step of developing formal recommendations for clinical actions based on the quality and quantity of the scientific evidence.

CPGs are most useful when they are based on a large number of high-quality studies, when they are developed in a way that minimizes the potential impact of subjective bias, and when their transitory nature and the need for frequent updating to incorporate new evidence are acknowledged. At present, there are a number of examples of CPGs on a single topic that were developed by different review groups that yield conflicting views of the evidence and contradictory recommendations to practitioners. Thus, CPGs must also be appraised critically with the themes of validity and importance in mind. To this end, a common set of quality indicators for CPGs has been proposed (Cluzeau et al., 2003).

In short, carefully conducted and current CPGs may be helpful with respect to the external research component of E^3BP, but E^3BP may lead to clinical decisions that differ from those recommended in a CPG. Again, a CPG should not be viewed as dictating clinical care but rather as a potential source of external evidence to be considered when using E^3BP to make decisions about clinical care.

E^3BP: A REALITY CHECK

We face myriad clinical decisions about unique patients every day in practice settings that likewise have unique requirements and resources. The calculus of integrating all of these variables with three kinds of best evidence for clinical practice sounds daunting if not completely impossible. Does E^3BP demand that we have the best available external, internal, and patient-preference evidence to back up every clinical decision we make for every patient we see? If not, what are the circumstances under which we should view E^3BP not just as a noble ideal but rather as something more like an ethical mandate?

These questions do not have easy answers, but the notions of honest (unbiased) uncertainty and clinical ethical reasoning provide a way to approach them. For example, there are many clinical decisions for which high-quality external evidence is not available. Although estimates vary, studies suggest that even in medicine, where strong epidemiologic research methods have been employed for more than 30 years, less than half of treatment decisions can be supported by the highest level of external evidence (Djulbegovic et al., 1999; Michaud, McGowan, van der Jagt, Wells, & Tugwell, 1998). There are probably just as many clinical actions for which external, internal, and patient preference evidence is equivocal—that is, no one clinical approach can be shown to be substantially superior to its alternatives. In such cases, competent and ethically responsible clinicians can readily justify decisions based on their own education and experience in conjunction with the progress and positive reactions of their patients. It is when honest and unbiased clinicians recognize that there is cause for uncertainty about the optimal clinical decision that E^{3}BP provides a very helpful tool.

Unfortunately, uncertainty is not a perfect guide to deciding when to use E^{3}BP in a more formal or explicit manner because everyone has had the experience of being 100% certain of something that was later found to be wrong. Barrett-Connor (2002) paraphrased Pickering (1964) on the essential tension between certainty and questioning that faces clinical scientists.

> If you are a clinician, you must believe that you know what will help your patient; otherwise, you cannot counsel, you cannot prescribe. If you are a scientist, however, you must be uncertain—a scientist who no longer asks questions is a bad scientist. (p. 30)

If clinicians recognize the need to review their patients' progress and their own performance in an unbiased fashion, to update their knowledge on a regular basis, and to question their subjective beliefs and assumptions, E^{3}BP provides a way to balance the roles of clinician and scientist.

The remainder of this handbook is organized as follows. Chapter 2 discusses how to turn uncertainty into the kinds of questions needed for productive and efficient evidence searches. Chapter 3 concerns searching for external evidence. Chapters 4 and 5 provide overviews of validity and importance, two of the most important criteria for determining whether evidence is sufficiently credible and strong that it could alter one's current clinical approach (e.g., Ebell, 1998). Chapters 6 and 7 show how to apply these ideas in appraising evidence from individual studies of treatment and diagnosis, respectively, and Chapter 8 describes how to evaluate evidence reports that synthesize findings from multiple studies. Chapter 9 and Chapter 10 discuss the validity and importance of evidence from clinical practice and evidence concerning patient preferences, respectively. And finally, Chapter 11 discusses what might lie beyond evidence-based practice in the future of communication disorders.

2

Asking Questions
About Evidence

*It is not every question
that deserves an answer.*

—Publilius Syrus, Latin writer
of maxims

The goal of E³BP is to reduce uncertainty about a clinical decision by using best evidence from external research, from clinical practice, and from a fully informed patient concerning his or her preferences. But how do we find best evidence in any of these three domains? The literature on evidence-based medicine suggests that successful searches depend largely on something that happens before the search begins: namely, on how questions about evidence are framed. First, this chapter discusses how to structure questions about external evidence and then discusses how the same format can facilitate the search for evidence internal to clinical practice and for evidence concerning patient preferences.

QUESTIONS ABOUT EXTERNAL EVIDENCE

The scientific literature may contain external evidence concerning a variety of issues about which a clinician might be uncertain, including the optimal protocols for screening, diagnosing, and treating a communication disorder as well as the factors that cause or contribute to the disorder and the prognosis for patients who are treated for it. In this chapter, we will focus on formulating questions about treatment and questions about diagnosis, the two most common areas of uncertainty for clinical practice.

Decisions About Treatment

Take a moment to think of a clinical decision concerning treatment about which you are uncertain. What information from external research would help you feel more confident in making this decision? Think about a question that reflects your uncertainty, and complete the following sentence: I wish I knew _____.

According to Sackett et al. (2000), a foreground question (FQ) is most helpful in structuring the searches for external evidence. FQs include four elements (in any order) that can be remembered by the acronym PICO: a type of *Patient* or *Problem*, an *Intervention* (defined broadly to include not only treatments but also diagnostic/screening maneuvers), a *Comparison* or *Contrast* to the intervention, and an *Outcome*. Note that in FQs about external research evidence the *P* component does not refer to an individual patient (you are not likely to find external research evidence about him or her) but rather to a class of patients or problems. As mentioned previously, the use of FQs in seeking evidence about a particular patient will be considered shortly.

Here are two FQs concerning treatments for communication disorders with their PICO components marked:

1. In *toddlers with expressive vocabulary delays* (P), does *focused stimulation* (I) lead to *significantly greater vocabulary gains* (O) than *no treatment* (C)?

2. In *adults who sustained severe traumatic brain injury (TBI) at least 1 year previously* (P), does *a program of cognitive strategy instruction* (I) lead *to significantly better job performance ratings* (O) than *no intervention* (C)?

Identify the PICO components in the following two FQs:

- *In preschoolers with profound deafness, are reading scores at age 12 significantly higher for those who received cochlear implants than for those who were not implanted?*

- *Does a delayed auditory feedback device result in significantly improved conversational fluency for people with severe stuttering as compared with rate reduction therapy?*

Now contrast the FQs above with the two questions that follow. Which PICO components are present and absent in each of these questions?

- *What is the most effective treatment for children who stutter?*

- *Is individual treatment better than group treatment for aphasia?*

These two questions are not FQs at all. Sackett et al. (2000) would describe them as background questions that ask for general knowledge about a condition or treatment. The first specifies only the *P* component (children who stutter). There is no mention of an intervention, a comparison, or an outcome. The second specifies the problem (aphasia), the intervention (individual treatment) and the comparison (group treatment) in general terms but does not include any outcome. Here are some more FQs. What are their PICO components?

- *Do expressive grammatical skills of preschoolers with specific language impairments increase significantly more rapidly when treatment is provided daily than when treatment is provided less intensively?*

- *Does the frequency of challenging behaviors decrease significantly in people with severe mental retardation who receive functional communication training as compared with those whose challenging behaviors are punished?*

- *Is the frequency of cholesteatoma significantly higher in children who had tympanostomy tubes placed two or more times than in children who received tubes only once?*

PICO components can take a number of forms, as shown in the previous FQs. Comparisons can be sought between different treatment programs or between multi-element treatment packages that have been modified to include or exclude particular components. Questions can be asked about variations in the intensity of treatment, in the age or time point when treatment was initiated, or in the sequencing of treatment components. Positive outcomes can be defined with respect to absolute performance measures or with respect to rates of improvement in desirable outcomes or rates of decrease in undesirable outcomes such as challenging behaviors or harmful effects of treatment (although potential harms of treatment have rarely been addressed in the literature on communication disorders to date).

Each of the PICO components can be specified to a greater or lesser degree. For example, *P* components can be written rather generally:

- *For adults receiving hearing aids for the first time*

- *For preschool children with vocal nodules*

- *For school-age children with fluency disorders*

Or more specifically:

- *For middle-age, cognitively intact adults receiving bilateral hearing aids for the first time following a sudden onset of severe hearing loss of unknown origin*

- *For otherwise typical preschool children with vocal nodules resulting in moderate dysphonia*

- *For school-age children with severe fluency disorders that have persisted for more than 1 year*

The level of detail regarding the intervention, comparison, and outcome components can be manipulated in the same way, which is good because it is impossible to know the optimal level of detail to include in an FQ about external evidence without knowing how many scientific studies have been done. After a few tries, it will become easier to build FQs at the appropriate level of detail and to modify them as necessary based on the amount of external evidence that exists.

Now that you can identify PICO components and recognize FQs, please return to the question you wrote at the beginning of this chapter. Is it an FQ or a background question? Which PICO components did you include? Take a few minutes to recast your original question about treatment to make it an FQ with the PICO format. Start by assembling the four PICO pieces that you need, and do not worry about constructing a beautifully worded question. As long as you have specified the PICO components, you will be ready to search for external evidence. Also, do not be surprised if you find it difficult to recast your original question to include the PICO components without changing it rather significantly. Remember that FQs serve a very specific purpose (structuring a search for evidence in a maximally efficient way) and that writing them is a new skill that will take some practice.

Decisions About Diagnosis or Screening

FQs are also important when clinicians seek external evidence about how to screen or diagnose patients. Determine which of the following are FQs about diagnosis/screening and label their PICO components:

1. What's *the best way to diagnose auditory processing disorders in school-age children?*

2. Is *the CELF Preschool-2 (Semel, Wiig, & Secord, 2004) more accurate than the Preschool Language Scale-4 (Zimmerman, Steiner, & Pond, 2002) for identifying preschoolers with specific language impairments?*

3. For *identifying hearing loss in neonates, is distortion product otoacoustic emission testing as accurate as auditory brainstem response testing?*

4. How *soon should speech production be evaluated following a TBI?*

5. What *is the accuracy of parental estimates of intelligibility as compared with the Fluharty Preschool Speech and Language Screening Test-Second Edition (Fluharty, 2000) in screening preschoolers for speech deficits?*

6. Is *a perceptual rating of voice quality as accurate as an instrumental assessment for diagnosing vocal nodules?*

The second, third, fifth, and sixth questions are FQs, and it was probably easy for you to spot their patient/problem, intervention, and comparison components. You might have noticed, however, that the outcome component for these questions about diagnosis and screening concerns the performance of the diagnostic or screening tool, not the performance of the patients, and that *performance* here always refers to accuracy.

*   Is *the CELF Preschool 2* (I) *more accurate* (O) than *the PLS-4* (C) *for identifying preschoolers with specific language impairments* (P)?

*   For *identifying hearing loss in neonates* (P), is *distortion product otoacoustic emission testing* (I) *as accurate* (O) as *auditory brainstem response testing* (C)?

*   ·What is the *accuracy* (O) of *parental estimates of intelligibility* (I) as compared with *the Fluharty-2 Test* (C) in *screening preschoolers for speech deficits* (P)?

*   Is *a perceptual rating of voice quality* (I) *as accurate* (O) as *an instrumental evaluation* (C) *for diagnosing vocal nodules* (P)?

Accuracy is often the outcome of interest in FQs about diagnosis and screening because a diagnostic or screening measure that fails to assign patients to the "right" categories (i.e., those who have versus those who do not have a disorder in the case of diagnosis, those for whom further assessment is or is not warranted in the case of screening) can lead to inappropriate treatment recommendations, inaccurate prognostic statements, and so forth.

It is worth noting that evaluations or assessments can be conducted for several reasons other than classifying patients. For example, if the purpose of an assessment protocol is to identify treatment goals for patients already diagnosed with a disorder, then the FQ might be structured to compare rate or extent of improvement in those whose treatment goals were selected on the basis of that assessment and those whose goals were chosen in some other way. In such cases, the FQ actually concerns treatment rather than diagnosis, and the outcome component for PICO would accordingly concern not classification accuracy but the treatment outcomes in the two groups.

QUESTIONS ABOUT THE OTHER TWO KINDS OF EVIDENCE

FQs can help seekers of external evidence narrow the search space to improve the odds of finding useful evidence. What about evidence that does not come from the external literature—that is, evidence from clinical practice with a patient and evidence on patient preferences? Although the previous literature has not addressed the use of FQs in this context, it seems clear that FQs can be very helpful in structuring searches for these kinds of evidence too.

Foreground Questions About Evidence from Clinical Practice

Imagine a clinician who is uncertain about whether one of her patients is progressing as rapidly as he should and decides to seek internal evidence in an effort to reduce her uncertainty. This clinician will face a very difficult task if she begins with a question such as, "Is Jeff's treatment working?" or "Is Jeff making enough progress in treatment?" Although both of these questions specify the patient and allude to the intervention approach that the clinician is using, the comparison and outcome components are missing. Writing an FQ that includes all four PICO components would outline a much clearer path to the information the clinician needs and the process by which she can obtain it. For example, "Over 4 weeks of treatment, has Jeff's rate of spontaneous communication attempts increased more rapidly than the increase that would be expected due to maturation alone?" Specifying the PICO components shows what the clinician needs to find out in order to reduce her uncertainty, making the search for evidence about this patient a manageable task with a clear endpoint.

Similarly, a clinician who is uncertain about the effectiveness of the particular treatment approach he is using with Janie might, pre-PICO, phrase his question in general terms such as, "Is Treatment A the best treatment for Janie?" The intervention and the patient are mentioned here, but consider how the clinician could immediately sharpen the question, narrow the search space, and clarify what he needs to do in order to answer it if he also specified the comparison and outcome. For example, "Does Janie's spontaneous use of new words in conversation occur sooner if they are introduced via Treatment A than if they are introduced via Treatment B?" Framing the question with PICO makes it clear how the clinician could use Treatment A for one set of words and Treatment B for another and then note the date of first spontaneous use in conversation in order to determine whether there is a strong advantage for one of the treatments.

Foreground Questions About Patient Preferences

FQs are similarly useful when there is uncertainty about a patient's preferences. However, it may take considerable time to ensure that patients fully understand the costs, risks, and benefits of their clinical options. In my experience, it is more common for busy clinicians to present the patient with the option that they would recommend than to invite the patient to express a preference among the alternatives; for example, "Jeff needs treatment, and I can see him Mondays and Wednesdays at 2:00." By contrast, using the PICO framework enables clinicians to lay out the available clinical options and their cost–benefit ratios and to solicit the patient's or caregiver's opinion about the best option given his or her particular circumstances and values (Straus et al., 2005). Such a discussion might be framed in the following way:

> Mr. and Ms. X, there are two major treatment approaches that might be appropriate for your son, Jeff, and studies show that they both seem to be equally effective in increasing the number of vocabulary words that children use. One of the treatments would require that Jeff attend a 2-hour individual treatment session 5 days a week for at least 3 months. The other treatment would require that one or both of you attend three 2-hour evening sessions to learn some specific techniques to use with Jeff throughout the day. After you have shown that you understand how to use the techniques, you would use them at home as often as you can, and you would bring Jeff here to the clinic once a month so that we can measure his progress.
>
> I have seen good results with both approaches in treating children similar to Jeff, and in my professional opinion, there is no strong reason to choose one approach over the other. So, the decision about which approach to use is up to you, although of course we will monitor Jeff's improvement carefully to make sure that he is progressing regardless of which approach you prefer.
>
> I'd like to answer any questions you have about these two approaches, and then we can talk about the advantages and disadvantages that you think each approach might have for Jeff and the rest of your family before you decide which option you prefer.

This scenario shows how the PICO format helps to structure the search for evidence about patient preferences in exactly the same ways that it facilitates questions about external evidence and evidence internal to clinical practice with a patient. It makes clear that the clinician will need to have organized the best available external and internal evidence before conferring with the patient and family in order to ensure that they are fully informed, in keeping with the ethical principle of autonomy. Specifying the expected outcomes of the approaches that are being compared can avoid misunderstandings about exactly what aspects of the patient's difficulty are the focus of treatment. In short, using PICO to frame questions about evidence concerning patient preferences offers a systematic approach to seeking this third, critically important component of E^3BP.

Now that you understand how to construct PICO questions, it is time to discuss how to find the evidence you need to answer them, which is the topic of Chapter 3.

3

Finding External Evidence

Believe those who are seeking the truth. Doubt those who find it.

—Andre Gide, French writer

Armed with foreground questions (FQs) about external research, internal clinical practice, and patient preferences, you are ready to undertake the search for evidence with which to answer them. Of course, not all evidence is created equal; we're looking for best evidence (i.e., evidence that appears to be valid [or credible] and strong [or important]). Chapters 4 and 5 provide an introduction to validity and importance, after which you will learn how to use these ideas in appraising evidence from external research (Chapters 6–8), from clinical practice with patients (Chapter 9), and from patients themselves (Chapter 10).

FINDING EXTERNAL EVIDENCE FROM SYSTEMATIC RESEARCH

Before you can evaluate the quality of evidence, you have to find it. It is relatively easy to find evidence from clinical practice with a patient and evidence on that patient's preferences because the search space for such evidence is local. But the situation is quite different for external evidence from systematic research, which comes not from your patient but from other investigators studying other patients in other contexts. For external evidence, the search space is global, and the amount of external evidence appears to be increasing at an exponential rate. The prospect of a massive search through hundreds if not thousands of publications is one reason why practitioners may be reluctant to search for external evidence. Fortunately, several shortcuts have been proposed (e.g., Sackett, Haynes, Guyatt, & Tugwell, 1991; Sackett, Straus, Richardson, Rosenberg, & Haynes, 2000; Straus, Richardson, Glasziou, & Haynes, 2005) that can drastically decrease the amount of time needed to find useful external evidence (see Table 3.1).

Table 3.1.   Shortcuts to finding current best external scientific evidence

1	Do not look in the wrong places
	•Sources without controls for subjective bias and conflicts of interest
	•Sources unlikely to be current
2	Search electronically
	•Use high-quality sites readily accessible via Internet, such as
	www.pubmed.org (abstracts and some full-text articles are free)
	www.guideline.gov (guidelines and guideline syntheses are free)
	www.cochrane.org (summaries are free)
	www.asha.org (full-text ASHA journal articles are free to members)
	•Obtain library privileges through an institution to enable remote access to additional databases with free full-texts (e.g., OVID)
3	Look in the right places, in the right order
	•Evidence summaries/syntheses from transparent, reliable critical appraisal by formally constituted review panels
	•Evidence summaries/syntheses from transparent, reliable critical appraisal by individual authors
	•Reports of individual research studies meeting quality standards reflected in critical appraisal tools

Shortcut 1: Do Not Look in the Wrong Places

The first shortcut in a search for external evidence is not looking everywhere. Remember that the goal is to find external evidence that is both up-to-date and of sufficient high quality that it could lead you to consider changing your current clinical approach, which among other things means that the evidence should be as free of subjective biases as possible. The potential for bias is one reason why workshops, courses, and other presentations are generally not good places in which to begin a search for strong external evidence (although they can certainly be helpful for other purposes). Subjective bias is difficult to control under normal circumstances, but when a presenter stands to profit financially from the sales of devices or other products to the audience the potential for bias to distort the evidence is very great. Many medical journals have policies requiring full disclosure of all conflicts of interest by authors of manuscripts (e.g., Flanagin, Fontanarosa, & DeAngelis, 2006), and requiring full disclosure by presenters might also increase confidence in the validity of their assertions. However, because it is not feasible to assess the validity of evidence presented in such forums, they remain a poor choice for those seeking strong and credible external evidence.

Textbooks are also not recommended places in which to begin a search for high-quality external evidence, both because of the potential for subjective bias and more important because at least some of the evidence they contain will be out of date by the time they are published. Like presentations and courses, books can be helpful for other purposes, such as introducing background information on a topic or demonstrating procedures or products. Furthermore, in some cases there might not exist any stronger external evidence than what books provide. But there are much better places to begin a productive search for current, high-quality external evidence.

Shortcut 2: Search Electronically

We need to search in the most current research literature, focusing on outlets for publications that have undergone a process of peer review. Fortunately, this no longer means wading through stacks of journals in a library, at work, or at home. A computer or a personal digital assistant (PDA) with an Internet connection can provide nearly instantaneous access to a number of reputable electronic evidence resources (e-sources). Once you have current evidence at your fingertips, you will apply additional shortcuts (discussed later) to rapidly zero in on the small proportion of evidence that is both relevant to your FQ and of high quality. So, if you already are comfortable using PubMed or another such source, you can skip the rest of this chapter—PubMed is designed for people who have not tried an electronic evidence search and might feel a little skeptical about learning how to do one. If you are one of these people and can arrange to sit next to your computer while you read the next sections, you will soon be able to start using electronic searches to identify external evidence from the current scientific literature.

Shortcut 3: Look in the Right Places, In the Right Order

As noted earlier, an enormous and rapidly increasing amount of scientific information is available. Gaining access to every publication related to an FQ is not necessarily helpful because few of us have the time to read, appraise, and rank all of the external evidence available in the literature. Several search strategies and sequences have been suggested as possible solutions to the problem of evidence overload, such as the "4S" hierarchy (Straus, Richardson, et al., 2005) in which the search begins with computerized decision support systems and proceeds in turn, and only as necessary, to evidence synopses, evidence syntheses, and evidence from individual studies. The approach suggested in this handbook is slightly different although the basic idea is the same: Begin your search at the source(s) most likely to contain high-quality evidence and only proceed to the remaining sources if you do not find a compelling answer to your FQ.

Summaries/Syntheses of External Evidence by Formally Constituted Review Groups

The best way to begin is to look for an answer to your FQ at one of several sites that provide the findings of review groups formally constituted to appraise the external evidence on a topic or question with explicit, transparent criteria and procedures to minimize the potential for subjective bias. A number of such sites exist, including http://www.guideline.gov and http://www.cochrane.org; new sites emphasizing behavioral and educational interventions such as http://www.campbellcollaboration.org are increasingly available. If a recently updated external evidence summary or synthesis is available at one of these sites for your FQ, your search for evidence might be finished nearly as soon as it begins.

The highly respected Cochrane Collaboration originated the idea of training groups of raters to evaluate the quality of external evidence by means of consistent and rigorous criteria and then to synthesize the findings into an overall summary statement; the focus of the Cochrane group is on health care interventions from randomized controlled trials. The Campbell Collaboration focuses on social, behavioral, and educational interventions, applying similar criteria to evidence from studies with other kinds of designs. Both sites provide free electronic access to abstracts of their reviews, which will usually be enough because your goal in gaining access to these sites is to be sure that you are aware of any new evidence summaries concerning your particular question. Only if an abstract suggests that there is compelling external evidence with which you are unfamiliar are you likely to need the entire evidence summary. In that case, your university library system may be able to help you gain access to it through their subscription to the Cochrane or Campbell sites.

Evidence reviews concerning some topics in communication disorders can be found at the Cochrane site, but its focus on evidence from randomized controlled trials automatically means that a great deal of potentially useful external evidence is not eligible for inclusion in a Cochrane review. By contrast, the titles of several reviews listed on the Campbell Collaboration site seem likely to be of interest to practitioners in school settings, but as of this writing, many of these reviews are in progress. Because it takes virtually no time to gain access to and search these sites electronically, I suggest spending about 7 seconds (literally) at each site when you begin your search for external evidence, making sure that you are aware of any major new syntheses of evidence about your FQ before you proceed.

A third searchable site (http://www.guideline.gov) also provides a way to let evidence find you (Sackett et al., 2000). This site is managed by the Agency for Healthcare Research and Quality (AHRQ), an agency of the U.S. Department of Health and Human Services. AHRQ compiles current guidelines concerning clinical practices for various health conditions based on evidence reviews conducted by expert panels. Panels may be convened by AHRQ or by other professional organizations to conduct comprehensive literature searches and to grade the existing evidence concerning specific clinical practice decisions. The resulting guideline statements (freely accessible in either summary or complete form) generally present a list of clinical recommendations, each with an evidence grade reflecting the panel's evaluation of the quality and quantity of evidence available to support it. Some of the guidelines link electronically to detailed analyses of the strengths and weaknesses of the evidence reviewed. Although the majority of the guidelines at present concern medical conditions, a surprising number address issues and conditions that are relevant to speech-language pathologists (SLPs) and audiologists. You can register at this site (again, at no cost) to receive a weekly e-mail from the National Guideline Clearinghouse listing titles of and links to the new and updated guidelines—a painless way to learn of any new guidelines relevant to your area of interest.

A recent e-mail from the National Guideline Clearinghouse (2006) alerted subscribers to a new type of document that will probably be appearing more on http://www.guideline.gov—a guideline synthesis in which the guidelines on a single topic that have been contributed by different organizations are compared and contrasted by a nonprofit health services research agency contracted by AHRQ. The guideline synthesis in question concerned otitis media with effusion (OME) and summarized the similarities and differences among recommendations from the American Academy of Family Physicians, the American Academy of Otolaryngology-Head and Neck Surgery, the American Academy of Pediatrics, the Cincinnati Children's Hospital Medical Center, the Scottish Intercollegiate Guidelines Network, and the University of Michigan Health System for diagnosing and treating OME. Although at present there are too few guidelines concerning communication disorders to warrant guideline syntheses, as the number of guidelines increase, this will probably become one of the first and best places to search for external evidence concerning questions about a clinical decision.

If you are at your computer, try accessing http://www.guideline.gov, where you can search for relevant guidelines by entering key words or by browsing by disease or condition, by treatment, by measure, and so forth. Each individual guideline includes a brief summary as well as a link that takes you to the complete summary should you want to examine the specifics of the evidence and/or the review process more closely.

It is important to note that the guidelines at http://www.guideline.gov include a disclaimer stating that the National Guideline Clearinghouse neither approves nor endorses guidelines. Guidelines produced by different organizations may reach different conclusions or make different recommendations—that is one reason why guideline syntheses should be useful as they emerge. However, it is worth emphasizing that reasonable people can disagree in their appraisals of external evidence quality and that for the foreseeable future we are likely to have more evidence with shades of gray than evidence that is black or white. If you find yourself outraged by the findings of an external panel that has reviewed the scientific evidence in your area of expertise and has reached conclusions much different from your own about the quality of the evidence, it is time to step back and consider whether you are maintaining the dispassionate, objective perspective that should be the foundation for E^3BP. If you are sure that your reaction is based on objective knowledge rather than on emotion, then a productive reaction would be a respectful discussion with the guideline developers or the review panel outlining the specific flaws that you have identified in their analyses or conclusions. The emergence of explicit criteria for appraising the quality of guidelines (e.g., Cluzeau et al., 2003; Lohr, 2004) should also contribute to increased consistency among recommendations from different guideline developers in the future.

ASHA and the U.S. Department of Education also are compiling and contributing statements concerning topics likely to be of particular interest to their members. For example, members of ASHA can gain access to a registry of clinical guidelines relating to communication disorders at http://www.asha.org/members/ebp/guidelines that includes guidelines (and some systematic reviews) that have been rated with the Appraisal of Guidelines for Research and Evaluation system (Cluzeau et al., 2003). Similarly, the Institute of Education Sciences of the U.S. Department of Education maintains a What Works Clearinghouse (http://www.whatworks.ed.gov) that focuses specifically on educational interventions with topic reports that describe the strength of external evidence concerning interventions and direct links to individual investigations. The What Works Clearinghouse includes a disclaimer with its reports stating that neither it nor the Department of Education endorses any of the interventions included on the site.

Your first stop at one of the sites described previously (or similar ones that are sure to emerge) might provide you with a recent synthesis that gives you exactly what you need—a clear answer to your FQ that is based on high-quality external evidence. If so, and if you have no reason to suspect that evidence strong enough to overturn the evidence in the synthesis might have emerged since the time it was prepared, then you may confidently call off the search and use the conclusions and recommendations from the synthesis as the external evidence you need. However, if you find no syntheses, or the syntheses you find conclude that the external evidence is equivocal, you may want to extend your search to find current high-quality external evidence contributed by individual investigators.

External Evidence from Individual Investigators

Individual investigators (or groups of individual investigators) can contribute external evidence of two kinds: reviews of results synthesized across multiple studies and reports of original research studies. A review of the literature that addresses a clear and specific question and explicitly describes the methods and criteria by which studies were located and selected for inclusion is known as a systematic review; recent examples have addressed such topics as the efficacy of eye exercises in optometric vision therapy (Rawstron, Burley, & Elder, 2005) and the optimal signal processing for pediatric hearing aid patients (Palmer & Grimes, 2005). If the authors of a systematic review take the additional step of using statistical methods to quantify the weight of the evidence across studies, the result is known as a meta-analysis; examples include a meta-analysis of clinical outcomes in aphasia (Robey, 1998) and of verbal fluency deficits in Huntington's disease (Henry, Crawford, & Phillips, 2005). Because systematic reviews and meta-analyses are derived from multiple studies, they generally provide more reliable evidence than can be found in a single study, although like any source of external evidence their quality must be appraised (see Chapter 8).

As mentioned earlier, Internet search engines or evidence compilers can provide an efficient way for evidence seekers to gain access to external evidence of all kinds. A number of these are available and each has its particular strengths. This handbook will acquaint you with PubMed, one of the most popular evidence compilers. Although others (e.g., Embase) cast a wider net for studies published outside the United States, PubMed's accessibility and ease of use make it a good choice for external evidence rookies. Accordingly, the next section provides a brief introduction to what PubMed is, what it does, and how you can use it to find current, relevant external evidence in a matter of minutes (or even seconds).

PubMed: Getting Acquainted   PubMed is a web-based system for retrieving information from the life sciences literature. It was developed by the U.S. National Center for Biotechnology Information (NCBI) at the National Library of Medicine. PubMed contains bibliographic citations from thousands of life sciences journals, including those relating to speech-language pathology, audiology, and related disciplines, some going as far back as the 1950s. It is easy to find PubMed without knowing (or remembering) its URL—enter http://www.pubmed.org or type *PubMed* into any search engine.

The best introduction to PubMed is the Tutorial at the PubMed site. The purpose of the next few paragraphs is to make you aware of some of the unique features of PubMed that will make your initial efforts to find useful external evidence efficient and painless. Once you have an idea of what PubMed (and other online evidence sources) can do for you, you will want to consult the PubMed tutorial or other sources on electronic searching (e.g., McKibbon, 1999) for additional tips.

Searches with PubMed   There are several ways to use PubMed to find evidence; we will consider just one tactic here. As with other search engines, the process of finding evidence on your FQ begins by entering a word or phrase into a Search box; the search engine returns information on the citations that have been flagged as being related to the search term by a human indexer. Because we lack a single, uniform vocabulary or taxonomy of communication disorders, relevant information might be indexed under several terms. PubMed addressed this complication through its standardized vocabulary system of medical subject headings, known as MeSH. MeSH terminology is used to categorize related articles, and by entering your search term (for example, "stuttering") into the search box of the MeSH database you will see the definition of your term that is used by the National Library of Medicine, as well as a list of related terms. (You also can examine where stuttering appears on the hierarchy of MeSH topics by examining the concepts that are superordinate and subordinate to it on the MeSH tree; the short, animated tutorials on the MeSH database will show you exactly how to use MeSH efficiently.)

By selecting Links to the word *stuttering* you can directly access articles related to stuttering in three ways. You can ask for all articles related to stuttering or for all articles in which stuttering is a major topic, or you can choose Clinical Queries about stuttering, which is usually the most efficient way to search for evidence.

The Clinical Queries section of PubMed was designed as a shortcut to clinically relevant evidence on a topic. At the Clinical Queries page, you can search directly for systematic reviews on stuttering. You can also search directly for articles on the etiology, diagnosis, therapy, prognosis, and clinical prediction guidelines related to stuttering. You can choose either a narrow, specific search, which will usually result in fewer but more directly relevant articles, or you can choose a broad, sensitive search, which will usually not miss many related articles but will probably return some that are not relevant to your question.

As mentioned above, there are several other ways to search PubMed for evidence, and if you explore the site and work through the Tutorials you may decide that you prefer more elaborate and user-controlled search strategies. But the route from a search term to MeSH and Clinical Queries is the most efficient and user-friendly way to access external evidence.

Saving PubMed Searches in My NCBI   My NCBI is a virtual locker in which you can store, keep track of, and update the various electronic evidence searches you run. Setting up My NCBI for yourself is free and takes less than a minute—simply click on My NCBI and register your user name and password. After that, your virtual locker will be open to you every time you sign in at PubMed, from any computer or location. Any time you run an evidence search you can save it in My NCBI with a name that you give it or the search terms you used; the system will inform you how long it has been since you ran each of the searches you have saved, and you can also request e-mails notifying you when new papers on the topic enter the PubMed system.

Everything you save in your My NCBI will remain there until you actively remove it. When you return to PubMed after weeks or months, you can go to My NCBI, click on one of your stored searches, and immediately gain access to the list of results, or you can select one of your searches and use What's New for Selected to see a list of the articles that have become available since you last searched. Of course, if you had selected the e-mail update option when you saved the search in your My NCBI, you would already have been notified of the new citations. As you can imagine, both of these features are extraordinarily helpful in the quest to locate best current external evidence for E³BP.

Working with PubMed Search Results   Regardless of whether you use the Clinical Query or another strategy, your search will result in a list of citations, most of which you can select in order to see their abstracts. Scanning the abstracts for certain words and phrases suggesting that the article contains strong evidence and is therefore worth examining more closely is the next step of "evidence triage," and you will learn more about this process in the remainder of the handbook. The growing movement toward standard terminology and formats for abstracts and articles concerning clinical activities, such as the CONSORT statement for treatment studies (Moher, Schulz, & Altman, 2001) and the STARD statement for studies of diagnosis and screening (Bossuyt et al., 2003), will make this stage in evidence searching even faster in the future.

When you have identified one or a small number of articles that look most relevant to your question, your next step is to gain access to the full text of the few articles that appear most likely to contain current best evidence so that you can appraise their evidence critically. If the PubMed icon next to the citation is in color, then clicking it will either immediately yield the full-text manuscript (which you can choose to read in HTML format or as a PDF file that looks exactly like the published paper) or will take you to an Internet site where you can get the full text. For other articles, the full-text version can sometimes be accessed via the Links and/or LinkOut options. If the full text of the article is available online, then you will see a statement such as "Full text available at ___." Clicking this link will take you directly to the article itself or to the aggregator offering access to the full text electronically.

There are a couple of reasons why the full-text version of an article might not be available. One is that the journal in which the article appears has not made the transition to the Internet age, although there are fewer and fewer of such paper-only publication outlets. Another is that the article was published prior to the point at which the journal began publishing electronically; many journals, including those published by ASHA, are gradually working backward through the years to make more and more previously published articles available electronically. In some cases, the full text of the article is available electronically but not for free—the aggregator charges a fee to retrieve the article. If you are doing your search through a university or hospital library system that has paid the requisite fee to the aggregator, then you will usually be able to gain access to the article at no cost. If you are working from home and have gained access to PubMed through the World Wide Web while not connected to a university or other facility's server, then you might be asked to pay for the article. SLPs and audiologists need to be vocal and persistent in apprising their employers and administrators of their need for access to the electronic literature in the service of E³BP.

Full-text articles may sometimes be available through other routes than the PubMed site. For example, ASHA members can gain access to full-text articles from ASHA journals published as early as 1980 via http://www.asha.org. You can use PubMed's Single Citation Matcher to get the information you will need to find the article itself (e.g., journal, publication date, volume, authors, key title words). In addition, some authors make their articles available on their personal web sites, so as a last resort to accessing a citation for free you can try entering the author's name into a general search engine.

Although electronic databases are more likely than textbooks to yield evidence that is up-to-date, they cannot yield evidence that is up to the minute. It may take up to 6 months (or longer) for a published article to be indexed and accessible in a database such as PubMed, so it is a good idea to spend a few minutes scanning the contents (and, if warranted, the abstracts) of the latest issues of any high-yield journals for your FQ. In addition, Straus, Richardson and colleagues (2005) noted that patients may ask you about clinical approaches that are too new to have citations in PubMed. In these cases you can use a general search engine to see where your patients are finding evidence and then discuss with them the extent to which the evidence is likely to be valid and important. As we will discuss in Chapter 9, a lack of strong external evidence on a clinical approach does not mean that it cannot or should not be considered, as external evidence is only one of the kinds of evidence needed for E³BP.

Your electronic evidence search is more likely to yield too much external evidence than too little. If E³BP is to be feasible, then you need to know how to quickly discard poor-quality evidence and focus on the high-quality evidence that should influence your clinical decision making. This requires you to sit in judgment on external evidence, rapidly applying specific appraisal criteria to weed out the evidence that you can discount without a second thought. All of the criteria that you will use to evaluate the quality of evidence, whether it is external evidence, evidence from clinical practice, or evidence concerning patient preferences, can be linked to the ideas of *validity* and *importance*. The next two chapters will discuss how these ideas influence judgments about the quality of evidence for clinical decisions.

4

Validity of Evidence

An Overview

*The truth is rarely pure
and never simple.*
—Oscar Wilde, Irish writer

You are probably most familiar with the word *validity* from your coursework on tests and measurement when it refers to whether a test accurately reflects the construct that it was designed to measure. Likewise, when we consider the validity of evidence, we ask whether it is likely to provide a true reflection or a distorted view of reality. This is not the place to ponder philosophical questions about the nature of reality and the status of our efforts to understand it. Interested readers will find a concise and useful analysis of constructs such as objectivity and subjectivity in the context of quantitatively oriented and qualitatively oriented research in Hegelund (2005). However, there is an important distinction to be drawn between evidence from external research and from clinical practice and evidence from fully informed patients about their preferences. Both external evidence from scientific research and internal evidence from clinical practice are based on empirical observations of the physical world that can be verified independently by other observers. Accordingly, for these two kinds of evidence, we can directly compare results across observers to determine whether they appear to be valid (i.e., to provide accurate reflections of reality). By contrast, evidence about a patient's preferences is inherently subjective; its validity cannot be verified by anyone other than the patient. Chapter 10 considers how to create conditions that will facilitate the ability of patients to fully understand and freely express their preferences among the clinical options available to them.

Discussions about validity usually focus on external evidence from scientific research, where a distinction is drawn between *internal* and *external validity* (note that these are *not* synonyms for *internal* and *external evidence*). Internal validity concerns the extent to which empirical evidence provides a true or accurate reflection of the patients, procedures, and settings that were observed. Internal validity is an important criterion for appraising both evidence from research and evidence from clinical practice with an individual patient. External validity (also known as *generalizability*) concerns the extent to which the evidence provides an accurate reflection of patients, procedures, and settings other than those that were observed. External validity is an important criterion for research evidence because we would like to be confident that a study's results would apply to patients on our own caseloads. However, when we examine evidence from clinical practice with an individual patient external validity generally is not a concern; the goal here is evidence that provides an accurate reflection of this particular patient, not evidence that would license confident inferences about other patients.

This chapter begins by considering the main factors that influence internal validity, first with respect to external evidence from scientific research and then with respect to evidence from clinical practice. It then examines the factors that influence external validity, which is most likely to be a concern when we consider external evidence from scientific literature.

INTERNAL VALIDITY

As mentioned above, it is important to consider internal validity when evaluating evidence from external scientific research and evidence from clinical practice. In both cases, the goal is to determine whether the evidence faithfully represents the true situation for the participants in a scientific study and for the patient in clinical practice. Some of the factors that threaten internal validity are common to both kinds of evidence, and some differ. We will consider a number of influences on the internal validity of external evidence first and then turn to several factors that influence the internal validity of evidence from clinical practice.

External Evidence from Scientific Research

The internal validity of the first kind of evidence needed for E³BP, external evidence from scientific investigation, can be compromised by a variety of unintended, uncontrolled, or unknown factors (known as confounders) that can distort findings and lead to false conclusions or inferential errors. One way to rapidly determine whether the evidence from a research study might be sufficiently credible to influence current clinical practice is to examine the study in light of the following factors: subjective bias, quality of measurement, research design, miscellaneous nuisance variables, and statistical significance.

Subjective Bias   Subjective bias reflecting personal belief, opinion, and expectation represents one of the most serious threats to the internal validity of external evidence. As was discussed in the first chapter, human beings much prefer information that supports what they already believe, and they may ignore, discount, or fail to notice information that contradicts their beliefs and

expectations. Because these subjective biases can lead to inaccurate observations, analyses, and conclusions, failing to control them can seriously compromise the internal validity of evidence from a study.

It probably is impossible to completely escape the influence of subjectivity
in research studies because they are always planned, designed, conducted, and
interpreted within the investigator's subjective point of view and value system. At least, however, we can minimize the potential for a single person's subjective knowledge or beliefs to lead to inaccurate observations by using the
tactic known as blinding, masking, or concealment. Blinding has received relatively little attention in behavioral studies but its influence has been well doc-
umented in the medical literature, where studies show that bias can affect even
observations that seem to be completely objective. For example, Sackett et al.
(1991, pp. 38–39) described a study (Day, Maddern, & Wood, 1968) of doctors
who were given the seemingly straightforward task of entering fetal heart rates
displayed on monitors into patients' charts. The physicians all knew the normal range for fetal heart rates, but unbeknownst to them the investigators
manipulated the monitors so that some of them displayed rates that were outside the normal range. The study showed that normal heart rates were
recorded more accurately than were heart rates outside the normal range,
which the clinicians tended to normalize, recording them incorrectly in the
direction of the normal range. Sackett et al. (1991) suggested that the clinicians'
expectations and hopes might have clouded their observations in even this
seemingly simple and objective measurement task. It seems plausible that subjective bias might pose an even greater threat to internal validity when the phenomena to be measured are complex and subtle, as is the case for a number of
communication skills. Likewise, when measurement has financial or other consequences, for example when it is required to obtain reimbursement from
third-party payers, the potential for subjective bias to distort the observations
is a serious concern.

So, one important factor to consider in evaluating the internal validity of
an empirical study is whether the expectations, beliefs, or opinions of participants, observers, or investigators could have influenced its findings. For
example, consider a treatment study in which some patients receive an experimental drug and some patients do not. If the patients know that they are
receiving the new drug, then their expectations and hopes might affect their
perception of their symptoms in such a way that they experience better outcomes than do the patients who know that they are in the control (untreated)
group. Because the perceptions and observations of family members, clinicians, and researchers could be affected in a similar fashion, the validity of any
findings that favor the experimental drug would be questionable.

Ideally, steps would be taken to blind anyone connected with the study
who could have such an influence, including participants, family members,
those responsible for identifying participants or assigning them to groups,
those who carry out the study procedures, those who record or code the data,
and those who analyze and interpret the results. The terms *single-blind, double-
blind,* and *triple-blind* can provide a general indication of the degree of concealment that was imposed in an effort to minimize subjective bias, although the

terms are used somewhat inconsistently (Devereaux, et al., 2001). In a single–blind study, for example, either the patient or the practitioner is unaware of which treatment the patient received. In studies described as double-blind and triple-blind, various other personnel involved in the study are kept unaware of information that could bias its findings. Although it might be impossible to blind the participants and clinicians to different treatments that involve behavioral interactions, blinding at least those responsible for evaluating progress and those responsible for analyzing data would reduce the potential for subjective bias to distort conclusions about the size and significance of any differences between the treatment groups (e.g., Altman, et al., 2001).

Awareness of the importance of blinding to internal validity has led to a growing literature concerning the use of active placebo controls for both surgical and pharmaceutical treatments. Active placebos (e.g., Edward, Stevens, Braunholtz, Lilford, & Swift, 2005; Herbert & Gaudiano, 2005) are designed to mimic a treatment not only in superficial appearance but also in as many other respects as possible to prevent patients and others from deducing the patient's treatment group assignment. In some cases active placebos have involved sham surgeries in which patients in the control group are prepared for surgery, anesthetized, and provided with the same postoperative care as patients in the treatment group, although they do not receive the actual surgery itself. Administering a drug whose action mimics the side effects but not the therapeutic effect of a medication under study is another example of an active control. Describing a review of antidepressant therapy in which treatment was found to be effective in 59% of studies with inert placebos but in only 14% of studies with an active placebo, Edward et al. concluded that "active placebos seem to make a big difference, at least in some cases" (2005, p. 611). They went on to propose an ethical framework for weighing the increased risk that active placebos may impose on control group participants against the importance of the scientific question.

As mentioned earlier, blinding is a challenging issue when the treatment condition consists of behavioral interaction between the clinician and the patient (Herbert & Gaudiano, 2005), but at a minimum those responsible for measuring progress and outcomes should be unaware of any information about the participants that could influence their observations. External evidence from studies in which outcomes were measured by unblinded observers would necessarily be viewed with more caution due to the threat that subjective bias poses to internal validity.

Quality of Measurement   Measurement tools and procedures are also important influences on the internal validity of empirical evidence. Two interrelated questions need to be asked about every measure used in an empirical study (e.g., Thompson, Diamond, McWilliam, Snyder, & Snyder, 2005). First, does it appear that the measure could provide a valid reflection of performance? This question concerns the measure's reported or ostensible validity (face, content, construct, concurrent, and/or predictive) for the purpose to which it is being put in the study. For example, norm-referenced tests are designed to rank test-takers relative to a normative sample. Such measures are

(margin handwritten note: good quiz questions)

typically highly standardized (i.e., their administration and scoring procedures are explicit, and examiners may be required to meet certain criteria before they are qualified to administer the test). Often, their manuals provide supporting evidence of their validity, such as the fact that they correlate with other measures of the same skills, and evidence that their results are reliable across examiners and/or over time. However, most of these measures are not designed to be administered repeatedly to a single person, so the validity of their scores after the first administration is usually unknown. Thus, this kind of test might be highly valid for measuring a participant's level of performance at the onset of a study, before he or she is assigned to a treatment condition. However, the validity of using the same test at other time points in order to measure the effects of treatment is much more questionable (McCauley & Swisher, 1984; Zhang & Tomblin, 2003).

At the other end of the spectrum are criterion-referenced and/or nonstandardized measures in which a patient's performance is compared not with a normative sample but rather with respect to achieving a particular skill or level of performance (McCauley, 2001). When criterion-referenced measures are designed expressly for use in a particular study, information on their validity may not be available. In appraising results from studies involving such tools, it is important to consider whether their apparent face or construct validity suggests that they are appropriate for the measurement task.

Even if a measure appears valid and reliable in principle, the validity and reliability of its results must be considered in light of its actual implementation in a study since errors during administration, scoring, or interpretation can invalidate its results. Ensuring that examiners are well trained, monitoring the consistency of test administration on a regular basis, and conducting inter- and intra-examiner reliability checks are among the steps that can boost confidence in measurement results. Thompson et al. (2005) noted that investigators should report reliability information for standardized tests as actually employed rather than relying on reliability coefficients reported in the test manual because the degree of variability in the study sample is likely to be quite different from that of the normative sample.

Research Design   The research design of a study is another factor contributing to confidence in the internal validity of the resulting evidence. As noted in Chapter 1, research design has been the primary consideration in evidence-ranking schemes, where the design known as a randomized clinical trial or randomized controlled trial is acknowledged as the standard when the objective is drawing causal inferences about average treatment effects in groups of patients suffering from certain kinds of disorders (Norris & Atkins, 2005; Thompson et al., 2005; but see Concato, Shah, & Horwitz, 2000, for evidence suggesting that other types of designs can yield virtually identical results to those from randomized trials). However, no single research design is optimal for all objectives and situations. For example, randomized clinical trial designs are generally not appropriate for studies of diagnostic accuracy, for studies of etiology and risk factors, for studies of treatment involving clinical conditions that occur infrequently or progress slowly, or for studies involving an experimental manipulation that would be difficult to justify due to the potential for serious harm (Higgins & Green, 2005). As noted by Norris and Atkins (2005, p. 1114), "Results of nonrandomized studies may be so striking that it would be considered unethical to randomly assign patients" as would be the case, for example, in "all or none" studies where all patients died prior to the discovery of a treatment but some or all survived after it became available (Meakins, 2002; Phillips et al., 2001). Finally, if there is no evidence from simpler and less costly studies to suggest that a novel treatment may be effective it may be difficult to justify the expense of a randomized clinical trial. In short, a study's purpose, the nature of the phenomena under investigation, and the historical background co-determine the type of research design that is most appropriate for it (Glasziou, Vandenbroucke, & Chalmers, 2004; Sackett & Wenner, 1997; Truswell, 2001); one design does not fit all studies.

There are many ways to classify research designs, and designs do not always fall neatly into mutually exclusive and exhaustive categories. However, there are a few key dimensions along which designs vary and knowing them will be helpful in judging whether the evidence from a study is likely to be internally valid. Additional detail and definitions of the various study design types can be found in the glossaries of the Centre for Evidence-Based Medicine (http://www.cebm.utoronto.ca) and the Oxford Centre for Evidence-Based Medicine (http://www.cebm.net). In addition, a more elaborated schematic of study designs (Pai, 2006) can be found at http://www.med.mcgill.ca/epidemiology/ebss/Classification_study_designs_version7.pdf

Experimental versus Nonexperimental, Controlled versus Uncontrolled

Table 4.1 shows two of the major dimensions on which study designs can vary. The first dimension contrasts studies according to whether 1) the investigator has actively imposed a manipulation on a situation in order to study its effects, or 2) the investigator's intent is not to alter a situation but rather to observe it in a systematic fashion. Studies with active manipulations are known as having *experimental* designs. Studies without manipulations are known as having *nonexperimental* or *observational* designs.

The second major distinction concerns whether the study has been designed to compare results from different participants or different conditions, or simply to report on the characteristics of a single individual, group, or condition. Studies of the first type are often called *controlled* studies because they involve a control group or control condition. Studies of the second type are referred to as *uncontrolled*.

Table 4.1 illustrates how many of the most common study designs would be classified using the dimensions of manipulation and comparison. Most experimental designs are also controlled, in that data from those who experienced the active manipulation imposed by the investigator (the experimental group) are compared with data from those who did not experience the same manipulation (the control group). However, Table 4.1 shows that experimental designs may also be uncontrolled. This kind of study may occur during the early stages of investigation into the safety and tolerability of a new drug, when it is administered to a group of volunteers who all receive it.

Table 4.1. Common study designs as they might be classified on two dimensions

Controlled comparison	Experimental manipulation	
	Yes	No
Yes	Controlled trial	Cohort
	Multiple baseline	Case-control
		Cross-sectional
No	Uncontrolled trial	Case report
		Case series

Note: The scheme is neither exclusive nor exhaustive.

Nonexperimental (or observational) studies, however, are not intended to alter a situation but rather to simply collect systematic information about it. Nonetheless, as Table 4.1 shows, nonexperimental studies may involve comparisons that are to some extent controlled by the investigator. In cohort studies, for example, participants differing on some variable(s) of interest are followed over time in an effort to determine whether they experience different outcomes. Cohort studies are not experimental because the investigator neither manipulates the participants' group membership nor alters the events that happen to the participants over time. However, because cohort studies involve a comparison between people exposed or not exposed to some variable they can thus be viewed as controlled studies. Other examples of designs that are not true experiments but do involve comparisons that are controlled to some degree by the investigator (e.g., Kirk, 1972) include case-control, cross-sectional, and correlational studies. In all of these studies, participants having different characteristics are compared, usually at one or a few points in time rather than over the longer time spans that typify cohort studies. For example, in a case-control study the investigator might select a group of participants who have a certain communication disorder (cases) and compare them to a group of participants who do not have that disorder (controls). In a cross-sectional study, an investigator examines the relationship among variables in a sample observed at one point in time, often by computing the correlations among them.

Finally, there are some designs that are not only nonexperimental but also uncontrolled (i.e., they do not involve a comparison group at all). Examples of these are case reports and case series that describe the characteristics of a single patient or a series of similar patients. Prevalence and surveillance studies, in which rates of occurrence of some conditions are examined in a sample, typically employ uncontrolled observational designs as well.

All else being equal (which it almost never is), the internal validity of evidence from controlled, experimental studies is likely to be higher than that of evidence from observational, uncontrolled designs. When observing the world and trying to draw inferences about cause-and-effect relationships, there are so many potential associations and factors involved that it is impossible to know which associations are true and which are spurious (e.g., Guyatt et al., 2000; Sackett et al., 1991). By using experimental and controlled designs, investigators attempt to demonstrate that they can control at least some of the relevant factors and rule out at least some of the competing explanations for the results. Although these two features are not the only important contributors to the validity of evidence, the ability to quickly determine whether evidence comes from experimental or observational, controlled or uncontrolled designs is one of the first and most important skills used in the critical appraisal of evidence for E^3BP. Following are some examples. First, decide whether the study design is experimental. Then decide whether it involves a controlled comparison.

> *Two clinicians work at the same facility and use different treatments for patients with a certain type of communication disorder. Clinician A prefers Treatment A and Clinician B prefers Treatment B. At lunch one day, they each realize that they are both using their preferred approach to treat five patients on their caseload, and they decide to collect information on these 10 patients for a month to see whether those receiving Treatment A have different outcomes from those receiving Treatment B.*

> *Is the design of this study experimental or nonexperimental?*

> *Does the study involve a controlled comparison or not?*

If you recognized that this is a controlled study, but not an experimental one, you are right. In this example, the investigators did not impose a manipulation on the patients; the patients were already undergoing treatment and the investigators simply monitored their performance. However, the study does involve a controlled comparison between the five patients who got Treatment A and the five patients who got Treatment B.

Take a minute now to think about how this controlled, observational study could be made into a controlled, experimental study in which the investigators are actively manipulating or altering some aspect of the situation so that it is different from "business as usual." One way to make this into an experimental study would be to actively control which patients received which treatment, rather than just studying those already enrolled. Clinicians A and B could agree that the next 10 patients referred for treatment would be alternately assigned (after obtaining their consent), the first to receive treatment from Clinician A, the second from Clinician B, the third from Clinician A, and so forth. This simple tactic would make the study experimental because the patients would no longer end up with one of the clinicians as they otherwise would have. Instead, actions by the investigators directly determine which kind of treatment the patients receive. Of course, this experimental study continues to involve a controlled comparison of the patients assigned to the two different treatments. Here's another example:

> *A clinician has developed a new treatment technique and has been using it for 3 years. He finds that his patients have excellent outcomes, and he volunteers to make a presentation about his technique at a staff meeting. He wants to include evidence that the technique is effective, so he pulls the files for all the patients with whom he has used it and tabulates their rates of progress and their outcomes.*

> *Is this clinician reporting evidence from an experimental study? From a controlled study?*

I hope it can be recognized that the kind of study described in this example is nonexperimental. The clinician did not alter his usual clinical approach but merely reported on it. However, this study also is uncontrolled because the clinician is reporting observations only on the series of patients he has treated with his approach and not on any type of comparison group. Take a moment to ponder how this clinician could make his study controlled and experimental so that his evidence would be stronger.

To make the study controlled, he might consider comparing results from his patients with results from patients treated by another clinician who has not used his new technique. To make the study experimental, he would have to actively manipulate which patients were treated in which fashion, which would obviously require that he plan the study before he begins collecting the data. The advance planning that is needed to conduct experimental studies makes them prospective, and the distinction between prospective and retrospective studies is another element of a study's design that is considered during critical appraisal of its internal validity.

Prospective versus Retrospective   The distinction between prospective and retrospective study designs also contributes to a study's internal validity. In a *prospective* study, the investigator states one or more hypotheses, identifies the kinds of participants and procedures that are needed to test the hypotheses, and only then recruits participants and begins collecting data. In a *retrospective* study, however, the investigator analyzes data that had already existed prior to the investigation, so he or she has no control over the participants from whom or the means by which the data were collected. It can probably be seen that experimental studies must be prospective; otherwise, the investigator could not have imposed a manipulation and observed its subsequent effects. But nonexperimental studies can be either prospective or retrospective. If the investigator did not assign children to be treated by Clinician A or Clinician B but simply examined data that had already been collected on the children treated by these clinicians, then the study design would be retrospective as well as nonexperimental. However, if the investigator set up the study beforehand to collect data from the next five preschoolers entering the caseloads of Clinician A and Clinician B (without influencing which children were treated by which clinician), then the study design would be prospective as well as nonexperimental.

Studies with retrospective designs are ranked lower than studies with prospective designs because retrospective designs offer no means of controlling for systematic and/or unknown variables that could have influenced the selection of participants, their assignment to the comparison groups, or their experiences unrelated to the study. In addition, retrospective studies make it difficult, if not impossible, to assess either the fidelity or reliability of the study's treatment and measurement procedures because the procedures had been conducted before the study began.

Randomized versus Nonrandomized   A final design feature that influences evidence validity concerns the means by which comparison conditions are created in prospective, controlled, experimental studies. The ideal means for creating comparison groups is known as *random assignment*. In randomized studies, the participants all have identical odds of being assigned to any of the groups, and the group they end up in is determined by random chance (e.g., by a random numbers table). Randomization is by far the best way to reduce the chances that the groups do not differ significantly before the study begins, leading to increased confidence that any group differences found after the study can be attributed to the variable that the investigator manipulated.

The number of studies in which participants are randomized to groups is increasing in speech-language pathology and audiology, but there are many studies in which comparison groups were created by matching rather than by random assignment. In matched designs, investigators try to create groups that differ only on the variable of interest by ensuring that they are comparable on other characteristics that the investigator anticipates might affect the results. The key word here is *anticipates*. Even carefully matched groups can differ systematically on many unanticipated and unrecognized variables (e.g., Plante, Swisher, Kiernan, & Restrepo, 1993), making it impossible to know whether the variable that the investigator set out to study was actually among those contributing to any group differences that were found. Thus, matching is a much weaker strategy than random assignment because we can anticipate and match on only a few of the potential variables that could differentiate any two groups of participants. Random chance is likely to be a much better constructor of comparable groups than even the most conscientious and insightful investigator (Sackett et al., 2000).

Of course, random assignment is not even possible unless studies are prospective and experimental. If the investigator has decided to recruit participants before the study, then he or she can assign them at random to one or the other treatment condition. However, studies can be experimental and prospective without having randomized designs, as in the previous situation in which the investigator observes newly enrolled patients entering the caseloads of Clinician A and Clinician B but does not randomly assign them to one of these clinicians' caseloads.

Miscellaneous Nuisance Variables   In addition to the threats posed by subjective bias, poor measurement, and research design limitations, miscellaneous nuisance variables that could systematically influence the results of a study can lead to invalid (false) conclusions. Every study should be scrutinized to determine whether factors other than the ones the investigators intended to study could explain its results. Such scrutiny requires that we think carefully about how the study was conducted and specifically whether the groups being compared might have differed systematically in any way other than the one intended by the investigator.

Imagine a prospective, randomized, controlled study of first-grade children at educational risk who attend a 2-hour after-school program involving free play under adult supervision, with a ratio of 1 adult to every 20 children.

Children are first tested with valid, reliable measures to ensure that they meet specified criteria for educational risk and are then randomly assigned to either a treatment group or to a control group. Children in the experimental treatment group are pulled out of the after-school program each day for a 45-minute session of individual tutoring, whereas children in the control group have their usual after-school experiences. At the end of 3 months, trained investigators who are blinded to the children's group assignment administer valid, reliable measures of reading and math skills. Results of blinded analyses show statistically significant differences in favor of children in the experimental group.

How valid (credible) is the evidence that the tutoring led to improvements in reading and math? The investigators of this study did many things right, but there is at least one nuisance variable that could threaten its internal validity. Specifically, because children in the experimental group experienced not only the tutoring program but also substantially more individual adult attention than did children in the control group, the observed benefits might have resulted from the increased adult attention, alone or in combination with the tutoring program. Any systematic differences between the children being compared other than the intervention itself are miscellaneous nuisance variables that weaken inferences about the effects of the treatment. To strengthen the internal validity of the evidence from the study, the investigator might try to make the experiences of the comparison group more similar to those of the tutored children, perhaps by providing comparison children with an identical amount of individual adult attention that does not involve tutoring.

Controlling for every nuisance factor would rarely be possible, even if we knew them all prior to the study. However, when we consider the internal validity of evidence from a study, we must examine it closely to see if there are serious nuisance confounders that could plausibly explain its results. If so, confidence in the validity of the evidence must decline—even if the design of the study were strong, its measures likely reflected true levels of performance, and steps were taken to minimize the effects of subjective bias.

Statistical Significance   Finally, it also may be helpful to think of statistical significance in connection with internal validity because a finding that is statistically significant has a greater chance of reflecting the "true" underlying situation concerning a difference between groups or an association between variables than a finding that is not statistically significant. For E³BP we don't need to delve deeply into inferential statistics or the debates over the value of the statistical significance testing (e.g., Meehl, 1997b; Rorer, 1991), but it is important to understand that the *statistical significance* of a finding is not the same thing as its *significance* in the sense of importance or impact. For example, when a difference between a treatment group and a control group is found to be statistically significant, this just means that the difference was probably not a fluke—that is, it would rarely occur if the null hypothesis (of no group difference) were true. In this case, the p value associated with the statistically significant difference reflects the probability that the observed group difference could have resulted (from chance variation) even if the null hypothesis of no group difference were true. A statistically significant finding with a lower p

value (e.g., $p = 0.01$) is less likely to have resulted from chance variation than a finding with a higher p value (e.g., $p = 0.05$), although no matter how low the p value there is always a chance of making a Type I error (concluding that a difference exists when in fact the null hypothesis of no difference is true).

On the other hand, when a difference or finding is not statistically significant, it is necessary to consider whether the power of the statistical test was adequate in order to avoid what is known as a Type II error—concluding that the null hypothesis is correct when in fact there is a true difference. Statistical power will not be addressed in detail here beyond saying that statistical power, p value, effect size, and measurement reliability influence one another and that statistical power should be at least 0.80 in order to interpret findings that are not statistically significant with reasonable confidence. In other words, if a study reports that a finding was not statistically significant, and that the power of the statistical test was 0.90, there is a relatively low probability of being wrong if we conclude that the null hypothesis is true. However, if statistical power is low, the validity of such a conclusion about the meaning of a nonsignificant finding would be much more doubtful.

Evidence Internal to Clinical Practice

When we evaluate the internal validity of evidence derived from clinical practice rather than from a research study, we are concerned with the same general question: Does the evidence accurately reflect the patient's performance and/or the factors that influence it? Although statistical significance is usually not a relevant consideration for evidence concerning a particular client, we can assess such evidence with respect to the remaining influences on internal validity: subjective bias, measurement quality, research design, and miscellaneous nuisance factors. Because the goal is to determine whether the evidence appears sufficiently strong to reduce uncertainty about a clinical decision, evidence from practice with a particular patient will be most helpful when steps are taken to reduce the potential for subjective bias, research design, poor measurement, or nuisance factors to lead to false (invalid) inferences about him or her. If the internal evidence has already been collected, then we need to recognize potential threats to its internal validity so that our conclusions and inferences are appropriately cautious.

Subjective Bias   Subjective bias can threaten the internal validity of evidence from clinical practice because it is difficult if not impossible to separate the roles of clinician and investigator (Yanos & Ziedonis, 2006). For one thing, a clinician may become increasingly sensitive to the nuances of a client's behavior as a result of increased familiarity with him or her. This phenomenon, known as *observer drift*, can affect observations by anyone who measures something repeatedly over time (Hollenbeck, 1978). A more serious threat, of course, is the inherent conflict of interest between the roles of concerned clinician and neutral observer. One approach to both of these problems is to arrange for periodic reliability checks so that the extent of agreement between the clinician and a different, hopefully impartial observer can be verified. If measures of clinical progress are derived from durable media such as audiotapes, then it might even be possible to blind the second observer completely (e.g., asking him or her to rate randomly ordered and unlabeled tapes that cannot be linked to a particular patient or a particular point in time). Showing that a blinded observer reaches the same conclusions as the clinician bolsters confidence in the internal validity of evidence from clinical practice and strengthens its credibility as an influence on decision making.

Quality of Measurement   The same considerations concerning measurement quality apply to external evidence and to evidence internal to clinical practice. The measurement tools must be valid for the purposes to which they are put, and they must be administered accurately and reliably. For evidence concerning a patient's treatment progress, norm-referenced tests are probably inappropriate because few such measures are valid for repeated administrations over the short time spans typically involved in clinical practice. In addition, global norm-referenced measures are not designed to be sensitive to the small, specific behavioral changes that are generally targeted in intervention with a particular client.

Instead, clinicians often construct and/or use criterion-referenced measures that focus on specific treatment targets but for which validity and reliability may not be known. Of the various kinds of test validity that have been described, face validity (i.e., the extent to which people other than the clinician view a measure as a reasonable way to capture the client's performance) is the most relevant for criterion-referenced measures.

Confidence in the results of criterion-referenced measures also depends on their reliability, but in this case the concern is not inconsistency due to bias but rather inconsistency due to measurement error. Generally speaking, the odds of measuring something accurately increase with the number of measurements that are made of it. How many measurements of a patient's performance on a criterion-referenced task are adequate to ensure reliability? There is no way to answer this question independent of the particular patient and skill involved, but the word *reasonable* is appropriate here, too. For example, no experienced clinician would conclude that a 2-year-old child had mastered the use of the plural morpheme /s/ after hearing him say "shoes" one time because at that age grammatical forms vary from moment to moment and from word to word. But how many times would the child need to use the plural form for the clinician to feel reasonably confident that the child had mastered the form? One way to answer this question is to think about the cumulative probability that the plural form could have occurred by chance over successive opportunities. For example, let's assume that the probability of the plural form occurring by chance is 0.5. If we observe the plural marker on just one word and conclude that the child has mastered the plural form, we would have a 50–50 chance of being wrong (or right). However, if the child uses the marker on two words, we can calculate the probability that this was a chance occurrence by multiplying each word's individual probability of being pluralized (e.g., $0.5 \times 0.5 = 0.25$); this means that we have only a 25% chance of being wrong if we conclude that he has mastered the plural form. If he uses the plural marker on three words, then the probability of falsely concluding that he has mastered it is halved yet again (i.e., 0.5 x 0.5 x 0.5 = 0.125). What is the probability of a false conclusion of mastery if he marks it on four words? (Right: 0.5 x 0.5 x 0.5 x 0.5 = 0.0625.)

Thus, depending on the nature of the particular skill being measured, it may be possible to estimate (at least grossly) the probability of chance occurrence to arrive at the number of criterion-referenced observations needed for a reasonably low probability that results are due to measurement error. Probabilities cannot be estimated in this fashion for all criterion-referenced skills, but the general principle of obtaining an adequate number of exemplars prior to drawing conclusions is an important way to increase confidence in the internal validity of criterion-referenced measures used in clinical practice.

Research Design   Some of the research design factors considered in discussing the internal validity of external evidence are not easily transferable to evidence from clinical practice, but many of the same ideas can be used to obtain strong evidence concerning the effects of a treatment on a particular patient through the N-of-1 or single-subject design. Indeed, Guyatt et al. (2000) placed the N-of-1 randomized trial at the top of their evidence hierarchy for making treatment decisions about a particular patient. As Chapter 6 and Chapter 9 discuss, the concepts of experimental manipulation, controlled comparisons, and randomization can all be used to strengthen evidence from single-subject studies. For example, in the simplest single-subject design, baseline or pretreatment levels of performance are contrasted with performance during a period of intervention (see Figure 4.1). This type of pre-post design provides very weak evidence that the intervention is causally responsible for any improvements, however, because improvement might have occurred even if treatment had not been provided. Chapter 9 discusses several other single-subject designs that can provide stronger evidence that a treatment is effective for a patient. For example, if there is reason to suspect that performance might improve even without treatment (e.g., due to maturation or recovery from injury), then the type of controlled comparison known as a *multiple baseline design* can be used. In a multiple baseline design, more than one potential treat-

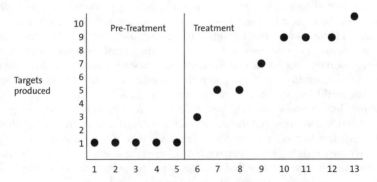

Figure 4.1. Results from a hypothetical N-of-1 treatment study showing the number of targets produced (of 10 possible) by a client over a sequence of five pretreatment (or baseline) sessions and eight sessions during which treatment was provided.

ment target is monitored during the baseline phase. After the baseline phase, one target is treated while the other remains in baseline. On the assumption that maturation or recovery should affect both targets equally, finding that progress occurs on the treated target but not on the control target can provide credible evidence that the treatment was effective. It is sometimes even possible to capitalize on the benefits of random assignment in single-subject designs, strengthening their internal validity even more. For example, a random process could be used in a multiple baseline design to decide which of the intervention targets will be treated and which will continue in the baseline phase.

It is not reasonable to expect clinicians to conduct formal single-subject studies as a routine part of their day-to-day clinical practice. However, when a clinician is honestly uncertain about the effectiveness of a treatment approach for a client, the principles of experimentation, comparison, and randomization can be used to obtain evidence that is sufficiently valid to reduce uncertainty about the best course of clinical action for that patient.

Clinical Investigation or Research Investigation? If the clinician decides to veer from the typical routine of his or her clinical practice, then it can be argued that he or she is approaching, if not crossing, the borderline between routine clinical practice and scientific experimentation. For example, the clinician might be interested in the effectiveness of a new treatment approach and decide to design a single-subject study in which the standard protocol is alternated with a new protocol in an effort to determine whether one approach is more effective than the other. As with any clinical action, the patient would have to be fully informed of the rationale for the experimental manipulation and the risks and benefits of contrasting the two approaches in this way before consenting to participate. It is worth considering the distinction between clinical practice and research activities because research activities are governed by formal procedures for ensuring the protection of human beings.

Regulation 45 CFR 46.102(d) of the U.S. Department of Health and Human Services (2005; see http://www.nihtraining.com/ohsrsite/mpa.mpa) defines *research* as "a systematic investigation ... designed to contribute to generalizable knowledge." Any effort to obtain internally valid evidence from clinical practice requires systematic investigation. It is the concept of generalizable knowledge that identifies the boundary of research activities. Guidelines provided by the Medical College of Georgia (http://www.mcg.edu/research/OHRP/BestPractices/Dist_Research.htm) suggest that determining who might benefit and who might be harmed by an investigation can clarify whether a protocol constitutes formal research with the intent of obtaining generalizable knowledge. Thus, if a patient is being studied in the course of clinical practice solely for the purpose of benefiting him or her, and if the investigation does not impose added burdens on the patient, and if the investigator does not intend to disseminate (publish or present) the information from the patient, then the activities would not constitute formal research.

If, however, the internal evidence is being obtained not only to benefit the patient but also because the investigator believes that it could potentially be disseminated to benefit other patients (e.g., the investigator is attempting to obtain knowledge that will generalize beyond his or her patient), then the research plan and procedures must be approved by the Institutional Review Board (IRB) of the clinician's facility. Clinicians in private practice or in facilities without IRBs should seek approval by an outside IRB. In either case, consulting with investigators who are familiar with the local IRB approval process will be quite helpful as requirements and procedures may differ slightly from IRB to IRB.

The IRB will review the research to see that the rights of the patient are being protected and that the requirements of informed consent to participate have been met. A great deal has been written about the elements of adequate informed consent (see http://www.nihtraining.com/ohsrsite/mpa.mpa.html). Generally speaking, informed consent requires that patients be aware 1) that they are participating in research, 2) that their participation is optional, and 3) that deciding not to participate will have no adverse consequences for them. In addition, patients must understand the purposes of the research, the procedures to be employed, the duration of their involvement, and the benefits and risks that can reasonably be anticipated. Finally, patients must be aware that they can discontinue participation at any time without penalty of any kind and should know how to do so. It is important to emphasize that the approval of an IRB does not guarantee that individuals will be protected from risks and harms. The investigator has the ultimate responsibility for ensuring that all patient contact, whether for purposes of research or clinical practice, adheres to the ethical principles of beneficence, nonmaleficence, autonomy, and justice.

A spate of publicity (Reynolds, 2003) concerned an investigation into the origins of stuttering that was conducted by a University of Iowa graduate student under the supervision of Wendell Johnson in 1939. This study occurred before the principles of ethical conduct governing research with human beings were codified in the 1947 Nuremberg Code, the 1964 Helsinki Declaration, and the 1979 Belmont Report (see Amdur, 2003). Unfortunately, its procedures violated every ethical principle.

In this study, children living in an orphanage were randomly assigned to either an experimental or a control group. Children in the experimental group were subjected to procedures that were intended to increase their anxiety about the possibility that they would stutter when they spoke. The principle of beneficence was violated as there was no foreseeable benefit to participants. The principle of nonmaleficence was likewise violated as children in the experimental group were expected to experience at least two immediate harms— increased anxiety and increased stuttering. The principle of autonomy was violated as children were not informed that they were part of a research project and thus did not consent to participate. Finally, the principle of justice was violated as the children's status as orphans led them to be unfairly singled out for the experiment. No attempt was made to enroll children living with parents who could have acted to protect their children's best interests, and even the orphanage personnel were not fully informed about the experiment.

The "Monster Study" of stuttering, as it has been called, provides a sad and overwhelming illustration of the importance of the four ethical principles in efforts to obtain external evidence. Exactly the same considerations should guide clinicians as they seek internal evidence concerning their individual patients, especially if they are using procedures that fall outside routine and accepted approaches to practice. Individual patients must understand the potential benefits and risks of experimental procedures, that they have the right to refuse them without penalty, and that only the clinician involved can ensure that their well-being and autonomy are being given the priority they deserve. Yanos and Ziedonis (2006) provided a useful analysis of the need to be aware of the potential ethical conflicts that can occur when a single person simultaneously occupies the roles of clinician and researcher; they note in particular the difficulty of avoiding the therapeutic misconception in which patients assume that any invitation to participate in a study that comes from a clinician should be accepted as it is likely to benefit them.

Miscellaneous Nuisance Variables   The internal validity of evidence from an individual patient can be compromised by a wide range of unanticipated and uncontrolled nuisance variables. Seemingly random day-to-day fluctuations in a patient's performance, for example, might turn out to be predictable in the context of medical, emotional, or other changes in the patient's life outside the clinic. When we scrutinize internal evidence from our patients, we need to be cautious about our inherent preference to interpret improvements as being due solely to our clinical actions and, conversely, to attribute decrements to outside influences. Thinking about the possible impact of extraclinical factors on performance is one way to ensure that we focus on the big picture of the patient's life, even when our clinical efforts aim at a relatively small portion of it.

EXTERNAL VALIDITY

All of the factors considered thus far operate to influence the internal validity of empirical evidence or the extent to which it accurately reflects results for the patients, procedures, and situations examined. When we assess the external validity of evidence, we ask whether the results would generalize, or hold true, outside the confines of the study from which they originated. Again, external validity is primarily a concern for evidence from external scientific investigations although it can also be thought of with respect to the generalization of skills acquired by a patient in the clinic to other communication contexts.

The most important feature affecting the external validity of a study concerns the extent to which the participants are representative of the larger population from which they are sampled. As noted earlier, a great deal of important evidence for clinical practice comes from nonexperimental designs in which patients are studied "as they are" rather than undergoing an experimental manipulation. For example, questions about the accuracy of diagnostic tools or the impact of risk factors on long-term outcomes cannot be addressed with an experimental design because people cannot ethically be assigned at random to experience a disorder or a risk factor for a disorder. For such questions, the best we can do is to carefully observe people who already have the disorder or are already at risk for it. For evidence from such observational studies to be externally valid or generalizable, the participants must be selected in such a way that they constitute a good representation of the population of interest. Ideally, this would be done by ensuring that every member of the entire population of interest (e.g., adolescent girls, adults with severe traumatic brain injury, 4-year-old children with phonological disorders) has an equal opportunity to be selected for the study and that no systematic biases influenced the inclusion of participants. In this sense, the benefits of random processes can apply to evidence from nonexperimental studies too—not in assigning people to groups but rather in selecting them for inclusion in the sample to be observed.

Any factor other than random chance that affects the likelihood that an individual is included in an observational study is a confounder that threatens the external validity of its results. For example, it is not uncommon for investigators to ask clinicians or facilities to refer patients to their studies. Although this makes recruitment much easier, there is clearly a risk that the types or severities of patients selected in this manner may differ significantly from the broader population. Studies of such clinic samples often yield different estimates than do community samples concerning the frequency of occurrence of a disorder, its severity, and the extent to which it is accompanied by comorbid conditions. To take one example from the communication disorders literature, clinic samples (including samples of children receiving special services in school settings) have suggested that boys are twice or even three times more likely than girls to have language disorders. However, in one of the largest studies involving a community sample of children with language disorders (Tomblin et al., 1997), there were only slightly more affected boys than girls—the ratio of boys to girls was 1.2:1. Similar disparities between community and clinic samples in the ratio of boys to girls with specific reading disabilities also have been observed (Shaywitz, 1998).

In addition to the differences that may exist between patients who are and are not receiving clinical service at a given facility, clinicians who are asked to identify potential participants for a study may consciously or unconsciously impose their own selection criteria and refer only those patients with certain characteristics (e.g., mild severity, good compliance, excellent attendance). Thus, results from studies of referred participants are less likely to validly represent the actual population of patients with a disorder than are results based on samples in which the entire range of participants had an equal opportunity to be selected for study.

Identifying every member of a population and selecting study participants randomly from among them will rarely be practicable. But the general idea of selecting participants at random is just as important in constructing samples for observational studies as it is in constructing comparison groups in controlled experimental studies. For both kinds of studies, randomization is an important safeguard against nuisance confounders that could threaten the validity of results. Even though true random selection for observational studies may be impossible, studies that approach this ideal are much more likely to yield valid results than studies in which participation could have been influenced by confounders.

Given the importance of randomization in selecting participants or assigning them to groups, you can understand why subject attrition from either experimental or observational studies can threaten the external validity of findings. Attrition happens when there are fewer participants at the end of the study than there were at the beginning. Unless attrition occurs for completely random reasons, there may be systematic differences between the participants who complete a study and those who do not, regardless of whether they drop out voluntarily, are unable to perform study procedures, or are lost to follow-up for other reasons. Full disclosure concerning attrition and loss to follow-up, as well as statistical analyses designed to determine the extent to which the initial and final samples differ, are important considerations in evaluating the external validity of evidence.

In addition to representativeness of participants, external validity also depends on representativeness of the procedures employed in a study, something that cannot be evaluated without a thorough and accurate description by the investigator(s). The word *replicable* is sometimes used to characterize the requisite level of detail (i.e., people not involved with the study should find enough information about the specifics of the study's conduct to allow them to conduct the study in an identical fashion). In addition to an adequately detailed description of procedures, evidence of (procedural) fidelity strengthens findings because it shows that procedures actually were carried out as described. Although it has rarely been discussed in the literature on communication disorders, generalizability of findings to other clinicians is another factor that contributes to the external validity of evidence. Of course, this requires that a study include multiple clinicians so that the consistency of results across different clinicians can be determined. If different clinical approaches or procedures are being compared, then it would be ideal to train all the clinicians in all the procedures and then to randomly assign them to the conditions being contrasted. Such a step would increase confidence that the findings would apply to any clinicians who meet the proficiency standards described in the study, rather than being attributable to the personality characteristics of specific clinicians.

SUMMARY

This chapter introduced the concept of validity, one of the most important criteria for identifying evidence that should influence clinical decisions. We will use these ideas in appraising the internal and external validity of evidence from various sources and for various purposes in Chapters 6 through 9. But first we turn to an overview of the other major criterion for identifying evidence that could alter clinical practice: its importance.

5

Importance of Evidence

An Overview

*The sensitivity of men to
small matters, and their
indifference to great ones,
indicates a strange inversion.*

—Blaise Pascal, French philosopher
and mathematician

Like validity, *importance* is a rather fuzzy concept with several possible meanings, but the phrase "substantive significance" (Levy, 1967, cited in Huberty, 2002, p. 233) captures the idea well. Value, effect, and amount or quantity are all terms that are associated with the definition of the word *substantive,* and all will be helpful as we consider the importance of evidence. This chapter will address four interrelated concepts that contribute to evaluating the importance of evidence: *effect size* (ES), *precision, practical significance,* and *clinical significance.* Each provides a slightly different perspective on the question of whether evidence should be deemed a great or small matter (in Pascal's terms), and keeping all four in mind will help us avoid mistaking the trivial for the important. We begin with the two quantitatively oriented indicators of importance: effect size and precision.

EFFECT SIZE

ES is a measure of a finding's importance that reflects something different from its statistical significance, although it, too, is closely related to null hypothesis testing (Rosnow & Rosenthal, 2003). As noted in the preceding chapter, a statistically significant finding is one that is unlikely (as quantified by its *p* value) to have occurred by chance or sampling error if the null hypothesis is true. However, we need a way to evaluate the importance of a finding independent of its

p value because small and trivial effects can be statistically significant, especially when the sample size is large (Rosnow & Rosenthal, 2003). For example, Cohen described a study of nearly 14,000 children that made the newspapers because it revealed a statistically significant link between IQ test score and height. Although the strength of the association was small (the Pearson correlation coefficient was $r = 0.11$), in this large sample the p value was < 0.001, and it was this "highly significant" value that was reported in the popular press (Cohen, 1990, p. 1390). Cohen translated the size of this statistically significant association into meaningful terms to show how small and unimportant it was—an increase of more than 3 feet in height would be necessary for a 30-point increase in IQ test score, or IQ test score would have to increase by 233 points for an increase of 4 inches in height. In short (no pun intended), when we assess the importance of evidence, we need to avoid being distracted by statistical significance levels. Statistical significance tells us that a finding is probably not a fluke, but no matter how low the p value, it cannot reflect the importance, or substantive significance, of a finding.

By contrast, the ES of a finding provides a way to think about its size or magnitude—that is, not just whether the null hypothesis is false but the degree to which it is false (Cohen, 1988). Although many ES metrics have been described (Huberty, 2002; Huberty & Lowman, 2000; Vacha-Haase & Thompson, 2004), they can be lumped generally into two (Thompson, 2002) or three (Rosnow & Rosenthal, 2003; Valentine & Cooper, 2003) main categories. For studies comparing mean scores from different groups (for example, a group receiving behavioral therapy with a group receiving pharmacologic therapy for aphasia), *standardized mean difference measures* such as Cohen's d (or simply d) provide a way to describe how much their mean scores differ. For studies designed to calculate the relationship or correlation between two or more variables in a sample (for example, the association between age and responsiveness to a new treatment), ES measures of *variance accounted for* such as R^2 or R-squared provide a way to describe the strength of the association, or the extent to which the value of one accurately predicts the value of the other. Finally, for studies that compare a dichotomous (binary) outcome in two different groups (for example, the number of patients who achieve normal speech recognition scores with conventional versus dynamic speech-recoding hearing aids), ES can be quantified with a measure such as an odds ratio reflecting the different odds of this outcome in the two groups.

Many ES metrics are standardized or scale-free, which makes them very useful in comparing results across different studies. However, there is no value at which an ES metric automatically becomes large enough to be deemed important. For one thing, ES is affected by the quality of measurement; if a study employs measures with poor validity or reliability, the resulting ES is unlikely to be meaningful (Baugh, 2002). In addition, Robey (2004) pointed out that an ES is an estimate that is always subject to some degree of error; thus an ES should always be interpreted in conjunction with its associated confidence interval (as discussed in the "Precision" section, p. 57). Finally, an ES has to be judged with reference to the nature of the variables being studied and the effects found in previous research on the topic (Cohen, 1988; Rosnow & Rosenthal,

2003; Thompson, 2002; Vacha-Haase & Thompson, 2004) as well as whether the research reflects an earlier or later phase of investigation (Robey, 2004). Consistent with the organization of this chapter, then, ES should be viewed as just one of several indications that the evidence on a question is important enough to warrant a change in clinical practice.

The merits of the various ES indicators under various conditions have been debated extensively, and readers interested in a more in-depth treatment of ES can consult a number of excellent sources (e.g., Huberty, 2002; Huberty & Lowman, 2000; Robey, 2004; Rosnow & Rosenthal, 2003; Thompson, 2002; Vacha-Haase & Thompson, 2004). But for E³BP we can manage reasonably well with a basic understanding of three conceptually simple and frequently used metrics for the size of an empirical finding: Cohen's d, R^2, and the odds ratio. Even if authors ignore the recommendation that all studies include an index of effect size (Wilkinson & the Task Force on Statistical Inference, 1999), in many cases it will be possible to estimate at least one of these ES metrics using the data that are reported. Although the following sections on Cohen's d, R^2, and odds ratios won't make you an expert in the nuances of the many ES measures, at their conclusion you should be reasonably confident in your ability to decide whether an ES is sufficiently large to be considered in clinical decision making.

Cohen's d

Cohen's d is a simple, accessible, and reasonably robust (Robey, 2004) measure of ES appropriate for studies in which the means of two or more groups are compared. For example, imagine a study of children with reading disabilities, half of whom received "distributed" tutoring for 15 minutes each day, and half of whom received "massed" tutoring in a single 75-minute block. At the end of the study, the average reading score for the distributed group was 85 and the average score for the massed group was 90; this difference was statistically significant at the $p < .05$ level.

Thus far we know that the massed group outperformed the distributed group, but how important is the five-point difference between their average scores? Does the size of this statistically reliable difference warrant a change to current practice, such that students being tutored on a distributed schedule should be shifted to a single block schedule? This is exactly the kind of question that the d metric helps to answer. The d metric provides a way to standardize the size of the difference between group means, translating the difference into standard deviation units that are interpretable regardless of the nature of the original scores.

If you understand the concept of a z score or a standard deviation (SD) unit score, then you understand the concept of d, which is nothing more than the size of the difference between the means of the two groups in SD units. A d of 1.0 would result if the average score of one group were one SD higher than the average score of the other group; a d of 2.0 would mean that one group's average score was two SDs higher than the average of the other group. For example, in a study of a treatment designed to raise scores on an IQ test having a mean of 100 and an SD of 15, respectively, a d of 1.0 would mean that at

Table 5.1. Means (*M*) and standard deviations (*SD*s) on an outcome measure for a treatment group and a control group

	M	*SD*
Treatment group	20	5
Control group	10	5

the end of the study the average IQ test score of the treatment group was 15 IQ points (1 *SD*) higher than the average IQ test score of the control group.

Calculating the value of *d* for a difference between groups in a treatment study is straightforward: All you need are the means and *SD*s of the two groups on the outcome measure (see Table 5.1). If the *SD*s for the groups are the same, you simply subtract the group means and divide the result by the *SD*. Table 5.1 shows the mean and *SD* for a treatment group and a control group on an outcome measure; the *d* value is $(20 - 10)/5 = 10/5 = 2$. This means that the treated group scored, on average, 2 *SD*s higher than the control group on the outcome measure—a difference that is certainly large enough to be considered important. Note that we get the same *d*, but with a different sign, if we subtract the mean of the treatment group from the mean of the control group (i.e., $10 - 20/5 = -10/5 = -2.0$), indicating that the control group scored an average of 2 *SD*s lower than the treatment group. In other words, it is the "absolute" value of *d* that indicates the magnitude of the group difference; the sign simply shows whether the group with the higher or lower mean score was used as the subtrahend.

What if the *SD*s for the two groups are not the same? Investigators are not unanimous on how to proceed in such cases (Grissom & Kim, 2001), but as long as the group sizes and *SD*s are reasonably similar, the pooled or averaged *SD*s from the two groups can still be used as the denominator for calculating *d*. Grissom and Kim described several alternative approaches when *SD*s from the two groups differ substantially. One alternative is to use the *SD* from the control group because the variability in this group is more likely to be typical than that observed in a more heterogeneous group of people with disorders. However, Grissom and Kim noted that even in randomized designs in which the two groups have similar variability prior to treatment, the treatment provided to one group might result in substantially different variability at the end of the study. Any time the *SD*s of the groups differ substantially, basing *d* on the *SD* of just one will lead to quite different values than would be seen if the *SD*s were averaged. For example, as shown in Table 5.2, if the *SD* of the treatment group were 10 rather than 5 (indicating greater variability), averaging the *SD*s ($[5 + 10]/2 = 7.5$) would yield a *d* of $(20 - 10)/7.5 = 1.33$, a more conservative estimate of *d* than would have resulted if the control group's *SD* of 5 had been used to calculate *d* ($[20 - 10]/5 = 2.0$).

Grissom and Kim (2001) made a number of suggestions concerning how to calculate and interpret *d* for groups with different *SD*s, including the combined use of *d* with ratio-based ES measures. An unstated implication of their paper, consistent with the perspective in this chapter, is that ES measures

Table 5.2. Means (*M*) and standard deviations (*SD*s) on an outcome measure for a treatment group and a control group

	M	SD
Treatment group	20	10
Control group	10	5

should always be interpreted cautiously and in conjunction with other estimates of importance if they are used to contribute to clinical decisions.

So, how big should *d* be in order to be considered important? As noted by many (e.g., Baugh, 2002; Cohen, 1988; Rosnow & Rosenthal, 2003), and consistent with choosing *p* values for statistical significance tests, there is no absolute criterion level at which *d* values become important because *d* is affected by experimental design and measurement issues as well as the nature of the phenomena being studied. Cohen (1988) suggested that *d*s of 0.20, 0.50, and 0.80 could be described as reflecting small, medium, and large ESs, respectively. However, he emphasized that in the early stages of investigation into a phenomenon before the relevant variables and measures are fully understood, as well as in the study of complex and multifaceted phenomena, smaller *d*s might be important and provide significant leads to be followed up in subsequent investigations. For example, if previous studies of treatments for a poorly understood communication disorder have consistently yielded modest (though statistically significant) *d* values ranging between 0.15 and 0.35, a new treatment yielding a *d* of 0.60 might be viewed as quite important even though it is below the level described as a large treatment effect. The *d* value of a group difference that should be viewed as important, then, requires a subjective judgment made against the background of ESs seen in previous studies as well as the study's methodological rigor (e.g., Vacha-Haase & Thompson, 2004).

***Practice Calculating and Interpreting* d**   Arnold et al. (2004) described results from a study of more than 500 children with attention-deficit/hyperactivity disorder (ADHD) who were randomly assigned to one of four intervention conditions: medication management (MedMgt), behavioral treatment (Beh), combination treatment (MedMgt + Beh), and community care (CC). Among a number of outcome measures, participants were administered a composite measure of ADHD in which lower scores represent better outcomes. The mean scores and *SD* for each group on this measure after 9 months of treatment (Arnold et al., 2004) are shown in Table 5.3.

As you see from this table, the MedMgt + Beh treatment group had the best (lowest) mean score, followed by the MedMgt, Beh, and CC groups. Some of these differences were statistically significant and thus unlikely to have occurred by chance. Specifically, scores from both the MedMgt and the MedMgt + Beh groups were significantly better than scores from the Beh or CC groups. We can quantify the magnitude of the differences between these treatment groups by calculating the *d* value for each group comparison. Let's begin with the first two treatments shown in Table 5.3: MedMgt and Beh. All we have to do is plug their means and averaged *SD* into the formula for *d*:

$$d = (M_{Beh} - M_{MedMgt})/SD$$
$$= (1.34 - 0.95)/0.535$$
$$= 0.39/.535$$
$$= 0.73$$

This d indicates that the average score of the MedMgt group was about three fourths of a standard deviation better (for this measure, lower) than the average score of the Beh group. This is a solid ES suggesting that the MedMgt group had substantially better outcomes on this measure than the Beh group.

By contrast, the value of d for the difference between the MedMgt + Beh and the MedMgt groups was very small: $(0.95 - 0.92)/0.505 = 0.059$, or about 6/100s of an SD. The size of this d value means that there is not a strong reason to prefer one of these treatments over the other based on ES alone, although there might certainly be other reasons (cost, feasibility, risk of harm, acceptability to families, and so forth) for such a preference. Again, an ES measure such as d is helpful, but it can never be the sole index of the importance of an empirical finding.

Now, calculate the d for scores from the MedMgt + Beh treatment group ($M = 0.92$; $SD = 0.50$) and the CC treatment group ($M = 1.40$; $SD = 0.54$):

$$d = (0.92 - 1.40)/0.52$$
$$d = -0.48/.52$$
$$d = -0.92$$

Based on this ES, there is a clear advantage for children who received the MedMgt + Beh treatment; their average score on the ADHD outcome measure was nearly a full SD better than that of the children who received CC. A difference of this magnitude would probably be viewed as sufficiently important that it should contribute to clinical decision making by practitioners charged with making treatment recommendations for clients similar to those studied by Arnold et al. (2004).

If you are still feeling a little uncertain about how to calculate d, you can practice by using the data from Table 5.3 to calculate d for the remaining treatment group comparisons, such as MedMgt and CC, or Beh and CC. You can check your answers against those reported by Arnold et al. (2004).

Table 5.3. Means (*M*) and standard deviations (*SD*s) on a composite measure of attention-deficit/hyperactivity disorder (ADHD) for groups who received medication management (MedMgt), behavioral treatment (Beh), combination treatment (MedMgt + Beh), and community care (CC)

	M	*SD*
Medication management (MedMgt)	0.95	0.51
Behavioral treatment (Beh)	1.34	0.56
Combination treatment (MedMgt + Beh)	0.92	0.50
Community Care (CC)	1.40	0.54

Note: Lower scores represent better outcomes.
Source: Arnold et al. (2004).

Next, we consider a measure of ES for studies that describe correlations within a single group rather than contrasting the means of two or more groups.

R-squared (r^2)

The tendency for scores or other measurements of two variables to change in tandem with each other can be quantified by a number of measures of association. One of the most familiar of these is the simple linear correlation coefficient known as Pearson's r. Values of r can vary between 0 (if there is no predictable linear relationship between the two variables) and 1 (if there is a perfectly predictable linear relationship between the variables, such that knowing the value of one of them allows you to predict the value of the other with perfect accuracy). It is easy to evaluate the strength or magnitude of the association when r falls at one of these extremes, but when the value of r falls somewhere between 0 and 1, which it almost always does, even experienced scientists frequently err in interpreting its strength (Cohen, 1990). Squaring the r yields r^2 for linear associations (or R^2 for multiple associations), a value that reflects the percentage of variation in one measure that can be explained or predicted by the other(s).

Imagine that an investigator examines a group of preschoolers who have been treated for speech delay and finds a correlation of $r = 0.5$ between their scores on an articulation test at the conclusion of treatment and the number of hours of therapy they received. She reports that the correlation was statistically significant at $p < .001$, so the association was probably not due to chance. But to know how strongly (or weakly) these variables were associated, we need to examine the r^2, which for an r of 0.5 is 0.25 (i.e., $0.5 \times 0.5 = 0.25$). The r^2 of 0.25 tells us that the number of hours of therapy predicts about 25% of the variation in articulation test scores and conversely that articulation scores account for about 25% of the variation in number of hours of therapy. Twenty-five percent is not a negligible amount of variation, but neither is it impressive since the bulk (75%) of the variation in either one of these variables must be due to something other than the second variable. Even when the correlation between two variables is $r = 0.70$, which is often viewed as a strong degree of association, only about half of the variation in one variable can be explained by the other, as shown by the r^2 value ($0.7 \times 0.7 = 0.49$). An even stronger correlation of $r = 0.9$ still leaves 19% of the variation unexplained ($r^2 = 0.9 \times 0.9 = 0.81$).

Just as was true with d (and any other ES metric), there are no absolute criteria for deciding whether an r^2 value is of sufficient magnitude to be deemed important. In fact, Vacha-Haase and Thompson (2004, p. 477) illustrated that a "medium-sized" d of 0.50 can be converted into its corresponding r value of .224 with a corresponding r^2 ($0.224 \times 0.224 = 0.05$); this means that accounting for as little as 5% of the variance between two variables could be argued to be a medium ES. Again, judging the weight of an ES can only be done by taking into account the circumstances, variables, and methodological quality of a particular study as well as the size of effects reported in previous studies.

Knowing about r^2 should protect you from the widespread tendency to overestimate the predictive power or importance of a correlation, even a strong one with a low p value. Finally, in addition to understanding what an r and an r^2 mean, it is also important to remember that a correlation simply reflects a statistical relationship between two variables—not a causal relationship. A well-conducted experimental study is necessary to determine whether one variable causally influences another. Our expectations might lead us to interpret a correlation between articulation score and hours of therapy to mean that increased therapy attendance caused improved articulation, but without an experimental study we cannot disprove alternative interpretations for the statistical association (e.g., that improved articulation caused increased therapy attendance, or that some other factor was the cause of both).

Odds Ratio

The last main type of ES measure that we will consider is based on comparing the probabilities of dichotomous events or outcomes in different groups. There are several types of ratio-based measures of ES that can be useful in thinking about the importance of evidence from studies with binary outcomes and conditions (e.g., patients either did or did not recover, improve, and so forth when they did or did not receive treatment, have a certain kind of genetic marker, and so forth), but we will consider only one—the odds ratio. A number of other sources (e.g., Bland & Altman 2000; Davies, Crombie, & Tavakoli, 1998; Straus et al., 2005) provide interested readers with more information concerning the interpretation of the odds ratio and its relationship to other ratio-based measures, such as absolute and relative benefit increases (for desirable outcomes) and absolute and relative risk reduction (for harmful outcomes), as well as the related number needed to treat (NNT) and number needed to harm (NNH). This section is designed to provide an introduction rather than a comprehensive description of the debate and discussion concerning the use of odds ratios and other ratio-based measures.

Put simply, an odds ratio compares the odds (probability/(1–probability) of an event or outcome in one group with the odds of the same event in a different group. Odds ratios can range from 0 to infinity. An odds ratio of 1.0 means that the odds of the event of interest were the same in both groups, an odds ratio greater than 1.0 means that the odds of the event were higher in the first group than in the second, and an odds ratio less than 1.0 means that the odds of the event were lower in the first group than in the second. For example, in a study comparing the odds of full recovery in patients who received treatment as compared with patients who did not, an odds ratio of 10 would indicate that the odds of a full recovery were 10 times higher in patients who were treated than in those who were not.

Like most ES measures, the use and interpretation of odds ratios have been debated (e.g., Bland & Altman, 2000; Davies, Crombie, & Tavakoli, 1998), particularly because they are easily confused with metrics that reflect probabilities rather than odds (see Page & Attia, 2003; Straus et al., 2005). However, in addition to several desirable mathematical properties (Walter, 2000), odds ratios provide a way to think about effect sizes that goes beyond group averages or correlations, bringing us somewhat closer to thinking about outcomes for individual participants. Even if an investigator has provided d or r^2, if information on individual patients and outcomes is available, it is easy and can be instructive to calculate the odds ratio for the outcome in the different groups.

For example, consider again the study of preschoolers receiving articulation therapy, in which hours of treatment and articulation scores were correlated at $r = 0.5$. This correlation does not suggest a powerful relationship between hours and scores overall, since the r^2 of 0.25 means that only 25% of the variance in one variable was accounted for by the other. However, one might wonder whether there are certain areas of the distribution of therapy hours or articulation scores at which the relationship would become more noteworthy. Examining the data from the 50 individual participants might show that 25 children had received fewer than 10 hours of articulation therapy and that 20 of these had below-normal articulation scores at the end of the study. The other 25 children had received 40 or more hours of treatment, and 5 of these children had below-normal articulation scores at the study's end. By dichotomizing the data in this way, it would be possible to compare the odds of a "good" outcome (a normal-range articulation score) in children who had received more than 40 hours of treatment with the odds of a good outcome in children who had received 10 or fewer hours of treatment. After setting up a 2x2 table reflecting this state of affairs as shown in Table 5.4, the easiest way to calculate the odds ratio is via the cross-product ratio: the product of cell a and cell d, divided by the product of cell b and cell c. For Table 5.4, the odds ratio is $(20*20)/(5*5) = 400/25 = 16$, which means that the odds of obtaining a normal articulation score were 16 times higher in children who received at least 40 hours of therapy than the odds of a normal-range score in children who received fewer than 10 hours of treatment. An odds ratio this large would suggest that a stronger relationship between these variables exists at some levels of treatment quantity than is suggested by the overall r^2 value. This odds ratio still does not provide strong evidence of a causal relationship between treatment quantity and articulation score—children who received more treatment might have had better prognoses to begin with. However, knowing that the relationship between the two variables is stronger at certain levels could usefully inform future experimental studies that would allow stronger causal inferences.

Effect Size in N-of-1

In a single-subject (N-of-1) design, the comparison of interest is between treatment and control or alternative treatment. But instead of contrasting results

Table 5.4. Articulation outcomes by hours of treatment received by 50 clients

Hours of treatment	Articulation outcome score	
	Normal	Below normal
>40 hours	20	5
<10 hours	5	20

summed over the groups undergoing the different conditions, in most single-subject studies the contrast is between a sequence of longitudinal data points from an individual patient during a series of alternating phases, in some of which one treatment is provided and in some of which no treatment or an alternative treatment is provided. Most often, the measures of performance are frequencies or percentages of occurrence during criterion-referenced tasks that are judged appropriate for repeated administration.

As noted by a number of investigators (e.g., Mahon, Laupacis, Donner, & Wood, 1996; Sheikh, Smeeth, & Ashcroft, 2002), randomization and blinding can be employed in N-of-1 studies to yield evidence with excellent validity. Indeed, when the question concerns the effectiveness of a treatment for an individual patient (in other words, E^2), Guyatt et al. (2000) placed the N-of-1 randomized trial at the highest level of their hierarchy of evidence strength—above systematic reviews of randomized trials. But until recently, the difficult question of how to evaluate the ES in an N-of-1 trial received relatively little attention. Traditionally, visual analysis was used to assess treatment effects (Horner et al., 2005), that is, when the level of performance, as integrated subjectively by the eyes of an observer across the data points, showed a noticeable improvement during the treatment phase(s) a significant effect was inferred. However, because different observers may have different thresholds for what counts as a noticeable change, there is increasing discussion about how to make these judgments of importance more objective. For example, Campbell (2003) used three ES measures in synthesizing findings from single-subject studies of reducing problem behavior in people with autism. One was the percentage of reduction of behavior from baseline or mean baseline reduction (roughly, the difference between the average during baseline and the average during treatment, divided by the average during baseline). Another was the Percentage of Nonoverlapping Data (PND), defined as the percentage of data points in the treatment phase that do not overlap with any baseline data point. The third ES measure, Percentage of Zero Data (PZD), is appropriate when the treatment objective is to reduce a problem behavior completely (i.e., to extinguish it); it simply reflects the percentage of treatment phase data points for which the behavior does not occur, once a single zero data point during treatment has been observed. The same logic could be used for treatments intended to increase a behavior to a specified level of occurrence.

Beeson and Robey (2006) described several variations of Cohen's d that can be used to quantify ES for single-subject studies. Based on their ongoing empirical analyses of ES measures, they recommended a statistic proposed by Busk and Serlin (1992, cited in Beeson & Robey, 2006, p. 165) known as d_1 for studies that include data points from at least one post-treatment phase (or A_2; note that this is not an active treatment phase) in addition to data points from a pretreatment phase (A_1) in which there is some variance. Interested readers are encouraged to consult Beeson and Robey for a wealth of information and examples concerning d_1 and related single-subject ES measures; it seems clear that the use of objective ES measures to evaluate the importance of evidence from single-subject studies is an idea whose time has come.

PRECISION

In addition to ES, another factor that contributes to a judgment that quantitative evidence is important is the precision of such evidence. The notion of precision acknowledges the sad truth that any measurement of anything is subject to a certain amount of error. However, when we use reliable measurement tools (i.e., tools that yield similar results under repeated administrations) and obtain a large number of measurements, we can be more confident that our results will be close to the true value, within a reasonably narrow range of possible values that is known as the confidence interval (CI).

Confidence Intervals

If you used a rubber band to measure something over and over again, your results could vary quite a bit depending on how much tension you applied to the "ruler" on a given trial. Using a metal ruler would result in a much smaller range of values because it is inherently more consistent (reliable) than a ruler with elastic properties. However, even measurements from a highly reliable tool are subject to some degree of error. For example, temperature extremes could cause even a metal ruler's length to vary slightly, leading to different measurement results. Similarly, factors such as fatigue or inattentiveness on the part of the person wielding the ruler could lead to different results on different measurement trials. Finally, measurement results also will differ if the thing that is being measured is itself variable.

The only way to cope with the inevitability of error, even when using reliable measurement tools, is to measure multiple times. If we measure something just once, our results could be far from the true value. However, if we measure it multiple times, the extreme error values should occur less often than values that are closer to the true value. As the number of measurements increases, the Central Limit Theorem (or "law of large numbers") predicts that the pattern of the observed values will gradually converge on an approximately normal distribution (the familiar bell-shaped curve). The average or mean value of this distribution represents the best estimate of the true value of what we are measuring, and the *SD* of this sampling distribution is known as *the standard error of measurement* (SEM) or *the standard error of the mean* (SE). When many measurements are made and they do not differ from one another very much (i.e., the range of values is small), the SEM will be small and even the extreme values will be relatively close to the mean (or "true") value. If the results of the measurements are more variable, then the SEM will be larger and the extreme values will fall relatively farther from the mean value.

Using the SEM, we can construct a CI around any measured value (or point estimate), defining the range of values within which the true value is predicted to occur with a specified probability. For most types of measures, the 95% CI is the span of about two SEM ($\pm$ 1.96 SEM) surrounding the observed value; this interval defines the range of values within which the true value would be expected to fall 95 times out of 100 if the measurement were (theoretically) repeated 100 times. Similarly, the 99% CI ($\pm$ 2.58 SEM) defines the range surrounding the observed value within which the true value would be expected to fall 99 out of 100 times. The narrower the CI, the more precise a point estimate is said to be.

Although the precision of a finding is another factor to consider in evaluating its importance for clinical decision making, just as was true for ES there is no absolute threshold for adequate precision. If a study represents an exploratory foray into a new area, a relatively imprecise finding with a broad CI might nonetheless be viewed as an important motivation for future studies with larger samples and/or more reliable measures. On the other hand, if the same imprecise finding were reported against a backdrop of investigations yielding evidence with greater precision, it would likely be deemed less important.

Readers interested in the details concerning how to calculate CIs for a variety of point estimates can get a good start with Appendix 1 in either Sackett et al. (2000) or Straus et al. (2005). In addition, a number of statistical programs can be used to determine CIs when raw data from a study are available. However, for most purposes in E³BP, it is sufficient to have a basic understanding of what a CI reflects, especially when investigators adhere to recommendations that a CI be reported for every point estimate (e.g, Meehl, 1997b; Wilkinson and the Task Force on Statistical Inference, 1999). For example, consider a study in which the average score from Group A was lower than that from Group B, with a d value (2.5) indicating that Group B scores were an average of 2.5 SDs better than Group A scores. Viewed in isolation, this impressive d might lead to the conclusion that the Group B treatment should be considered for use in clinical practice. However, knowing that the 95% CI surrounding this d ranged from -0.5 to 3.0 would lead to quite a different conclusion, because the true ES could have fallen anywhere between a difference in favor of Group A ($d = -0.5$) to an even larger difference in favor of Group B ($d = 3.0$). With a range of possible values this wide, the evidence from this study would not be viewed as important enough to cause clinicians currently using Treatment A to consider adopting Treatment B instead. If the 95% CI for the d of 2.5 ranged from 2.25 to 2.75, on the other hand, there would be more than ample reason for those using Treatment A to consider altering their clinical approach.

Forest Plots

When several studies of a question have been conducted, a visual display of their ESs and surrounding CIs (known as a *forest plot*) is an extraordinarily helpful tool in gauging the overall importance of their findings (Lewis & Clarke, 2001). Comparing the CIs for findings from multiple studies is a useful reminder that strong evidence requires consistency, convergence, and replication and that the importance of a finding can never be adduced from a single study (Meehl, 1992). Indeed, comparing CIs across studies is the basis for meta-analyses, which occupy the upper rungs of most schemes for ranking the evidence on a question.

Meta-analyses are described in more detail in Chapter 8, but examining a forest plot here will illustrate the value of considering both ES and precision in

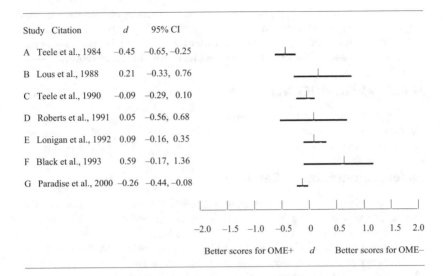

Figure 5.1. A sample forest plot constructed using values of *d* and 95% confidence intervals (CI) reported by Casby (2001, Table 2, p. 75) for seven studies comparing receptive vocabulary scores from children with (OME+) and without (OME−) histories of otitis media with effusion.

evaluating the importance of evidence. In a forest plot, ESs and associated CIs from multiple studies are graphed on a common scale. When the ES measure is *d*, for example (Figure 5.1), the horizontal axis of the scale might range from *d* values of −2.5 to 2.5, with the midpoint of the scale corresponding to a *d* value of 0 (indicating no difference in the means of the groups being compared). Each study's *d* with its associated CI is then graphed on this scale, making the distinction between ES and precision easy to see.

The forest plot in Figure 5.1 was constructed using *d* and CI values from among those reported by Casby (2001) for studies comparing receptive vocabulary scores in children with and without histories of otitis media with effusion (OME+ and OME−, respectively). As you can see, Study F reported the biggest difference in favor of the OME− children, with a *d* of 0.59 indicating that the average score of OME− children was slightly more than one half of an *SD* higher than the average score of OME+ children. However, the 95% CI around the *d* from this study ranged from −0.17 to 1.36—meaning that the "true" difference could actually have been in favor of the OME+ children. By contrast, Study G yielded a *d* value of −0.26 with a 95% CI ranging from −0.08 to −0.44. Although its *d* value is smaller, the narrower CI from Study G and the fact that the CI does not cross the *d* of 0 (which would mean that the CI included the possibility that there was no group difference at all) enables more confidence in its finding of a small difference in favor of the OME+ children. Although this small advantage for children with histories of OME might challenge many people's beliefs, the precision of this evidence suggests that it should be considered carefully, although the disparity of CIs shown in Figure 5.1 shows that this set of studies does not enable a confident conclusion about the relationship of OME and receptive vocabulary.

As noted earlier, ES and precision are two of the more quantitative factors that contribute to a judgment that evidence is sufficiently important to warrant a change in clinical practice. Next we consider two additional concepts that can be used in evaluating the importance of evidence for clinical decisions.

PRACTICAL SIGNIFICANCE

Although practical significance has been defined in a variety of ways and has sometimes been used as a synonym for ES, it is useful to think about the practical significance of a piece of evidence as a separate aspect of its importance.

Evidence from External Research

Consistent with the definition of the word *practical* is our examination of the practical significance of a finding from external scientific research when we evaluate its usefulness, or practical application, for the real world of routine clinical practice. The phrase "Patient-Oriented Evidence that Matters (POEMs; Shaughnessy & Slawson, 1997; Slawson & Shaughnessy, 2000; see also Ebell, 1998) captures the idea of practical significance rather well because it emphasizes that evidence is valuable to the extent that it could really make a difference to patient care. The notion of the minimal clinically important difference (MCID; Jaeschke, Singer, & Guyatt, 1989, cited in Man-Son-Hing et al., 2002, p. 475) is clearly relevant here; as defined by Man-Son-Hing et al., the MCID is "the smallest treatment efficacy that would lead to a change in a patient's management" (p. 469).

The idea of practical significance can also be related to the distinction between evidence of treatment effects (or treatment efficacy) and evidence of treatment effectiveness. Evidence of treatment efficacy is often defined as evidence concerning the impact of a treatment that is administered under well-controlled and therefore necessarily somewhat artificial experimental conditions. Evidence of treatment effectiveness, by contrast, refers to evidence concerning the impact of a treatment as it is actually administered in the far less controlled "real world" of clinical practice. The efficacy-effectiveness distinction also relates to the distinction between earlier and later stages or phases of applied research, with the typical progression being from early-stage findings that are obtained in the laboratory to later stages of investigation to determine whether the findings are also seen in more natural contexts (see Robey, 2004). The phrase "bench-to-bedside" is sometimes used in medicine to capture the same idea: that results found in the laboratory (at the bench) have to be tested in the world where clinicians will actually apply them (at the bedside).

New treatments usually appear more powerful when they are applied in the laboratory than when they are applied in everyday clinical practice. For example, an early-stage study of a new treatment for stuttering might involve carefully trained clinicians and clients who meet specific inclusion and exclusion criteria. Noticeable improvements in fluency for those undergoing the new treatment would suggest that it is efficacious in this well-controlled situation. However, when the treatment is applied by clinicians who have not received specialized training to the diverse range of clients on their caseloads, its impact might be less striking. In such a case, a study of the treatment's effectiveness might reveal that its practical significance is not as great as might have been hoped based on the early-stage results.

Although the progression in applied research often proceeds from the laboratory to the real world, there are many cases in which observations from clinical practice form the basis for subsequent studies in better-controlled contexts. For example, the realization that some patients were far better able to access words while singing than while attempting to speak provided the impetus for the aphasia treatment approach known as Melodic Intonation Therapy (Sparks, Helm & Albert, 1974, cited in Sparks, 1981), which was adopted by many practitioners before information on its efficacy under carefully controlled conditions was available. However, just as efficacy in contrived contexts might not translate directly into effectiveness in practice, effects observed by practitioners in the real world might not be as large when they are studied so as to control for subjective bias and other potential confounders. Regardless of the direction in which investigation of an intervention proceeds, its practical significance should ultimately be judged according to the context(s) in which it will actually be used.

Evidence from Clinical Practice

Practical significance is also an important consideration in gauging the importance of E^2, evidence internal to clinical practice with an individual client, most obviously when progress is measured only within the confines of the therapy session. Thinking about practical significance is a reminder of the need to evaluate the impact of treatment on the client's ability to take part in society, an idea that resonates with the International Classification of Functioning, Disability and Health of the World Health Organization (http://www3.who.int/icf/icftemplate.cfm).

Obtaining evidence on whether patients generalize their newly acquired skills to real-world contexts is one direct way to gauge the practical significance of internal evidence. Assessing progress by measuring so-called functional outcomes that are intended to directly reflect the patient's ability to function outside the clinical environment is another. Finally, social validity measures (e.g., Campbell & Dollaghan, 1992) can also contribute to judging the practical significance of changes in performance, in that an effect large enough to be noticed by naive observers might well be viewed as more important than a change that is imperceptible to the average person, even though it can be measured in the laboratory or clinic.

Finally, the practical significance of a patient's progress has sometimes been defined as clinical significance:

> Clinical significance is routinely defined as returning to normal functioning. Although for some disorders this may be too stringent a criterion, it is based on the assumption that consumers enter therapy expecting that their presenting problems will be solved. Even in cases in which this criterion is too strin-

gent, the scientific community, as well as consumers . . . still want to know how often normal functioning is attained. (Jacobson, Roberts, Berns, & McGlinchey, 1999, p. 300)

Atkins, Bedics, McGlinchey, and Beauchaine (2005) described several approaches to measuring clinically significant effects of therapy when defined in this fashion. All involve specifying a threshold for normal-range perform-ance based on normative expectations and defining clinically significant change only when a client enters or re-enters the normal range (see also Campbell, Dol-laghan, Janosky, & Adelson, in press). This definition of clinical significance depends on valid and reliable measures from representative normative samples as well as controls for the possibility that regression to the mean may be respon-sible for apparent improvements over repeated testing. When these conditions are met, comparing the extent or rate of change observed in a particular client (for E^2) or in a group of clients reported in a study (for E^1) to that expected of normal peers can provide another helpful view of the importance of evidence.

SUMMARY

This chapter addressed several ways of judging whether evidence should be viewed as important, including quantitatively oriented indicators such as effect size and precision as well as more subjective judgments such as practical and clinical significance. Whether the evidence comes from systematic scien-tific research or from practice with an individual patient, considering its impor-tance along these various dimensions is another key factor in deciding whether the evidence should affect current clinical practice.

6

Appraising Treatment Evidence

Since clinical experience consists of anecdotal impressions ... it is unavoidably a mixture of truths, half-truths, and falsehoods. The scientific method is the only known way to distinguish these ....

—Paul E. Meehl, American psychologist (1997b, p. 91)

Becoming certified as a speech-language pathologist or an audiologist in the United States requires "knowledge of research" (American Speech-Language-Hearing Association, 2006) and "experience in relating research to clinical practice" (American Speech-Language-Hearing Association, 2005b). However, some kinds of research are more relevant than others for addressing foreground questions (FQs) about clinical practice, and for evidence-based practice (E³BP) the applied research literature is a more likely source of external evidence than the basic research literature. The reason for this can be found in Table 6.1, which shows that although basic and applied research share many fundamental characteristics, they differ in purpose: basic research aims to increase human knowledge, and applied research aims to improve the human condition. Given that the purpose of E³BP is to improve a client's condition, useful external evidence is more likely to be found in studies with an applied research focus than in studies with a basic research focus.

This does not mean that basic research findings and theoretical considerations are necessarily irrelevant to applied questions; it just means that their

Table 6.1. Some comparisons between basic research and applied research

	Basic research	Applied research
Goals	Understanding, prediction	Understanding, prediction
Purpose	Increase human knowledge	Improve human condition
Philosophy	Realism	Realism
Method	Scientific	Scientific
Potentially relevant to	Human condition	Human knowledge

relevance has to be tested rather than assumed. History provides many examples of ineffective or harmful clinical practices that were based on accepted theories, and likewise of beneficial clinical practices that were discovered before there were theoretical explanations for them (e.g., Meehl, 1997a; Sackett, Haynes, Guyatt, & Tugwell, 1991). Accordingly, a strong theoretical rationale is more of an advantage than a prerequisite to high-quality external evidence for E³BP, and critical appraisal does not require familiarity with the latest theories (Evidence-Based Medicine Working Group, 1992). In addition, because untested theoretical claims about the clinical implications of findings suffer from all of the weaknesses associated with other forms of expert opinion, they will rarely represent the current best external evidence needed for E³BP.

To appraise external evidence for E³BP, we will use a systematic, structured approach that focuses on a relatively small number of key questions about validity and importance that often can be answered reasonably quickly. Sackett and colleagues (2000) and Straus, Richardson, Glasziou, & Haynes, 2005) described a one-page form known as a CAT (Critically Appraised Topic) for summarizing the current best external evidence for answering an FQ and synthesizing the results into a clinical bottom line. The CAT framework (see the free "CAT-maker" available at http://www.cebm. uputoronto.ca) has much in common with other systems for evaluating external evidence, such as the Scottish Intercollegiate Guidelines Network (SIGN; http://www.sign.ac.uk) checklists, and for reporting evidence, such as the Consolidated Standards of Reporting Trials (CONSORT) statement (e.g., Altman et al., 2001; Begg et al., 1996; Moher, Schulz, & Altman, 2001). However, because the focus in medicine is often limited to evidence from one or more randomized clinical trials, and because behavioral scientists such as speech-language pathologists (SLPs) and audiologists may be relatively unfamiliar with the process of critical appraisal as it is used in medicine, this handbook provides separate forms that are specific to the type of external evidence being appraised: a form to guide critical appraisal of treatment evidence (CATE), a form to guide critical appraisal of diagnosis/screening evidence (CADE, Chapter 7), and a form to guide critical appraisal of evidence from a systematic review or meta-analysis (CASM, Chapter 8). All three forms are intended to be used flexibly, and readers may discover their own ways of adapting them for maximal utility in appraising external evidence from individual studies. Note that there are several features that the CATE, CADE, and CASM forms share.

First, each form is designed for a single source of external evidence: a treatment study (CATE), a diagnostic study (CADE), or a systematic review or meta-analysis (CASM). Because the goal is a concise review of the strengths and weaknesses of the evidence, each form is designed to be just one page long.

CATEs, CADEs, and CASMs begin with spaces for noting who conducted the appraisal, when it was conducted, and the citation for the evidence being appraised so that it can be located easily at a later date. Specific words and phrases that led to the evidence source can be noted here as well and may be useful in subsequent searches.

The next section of each form is for specifying the FQs addressed by the evidence, followed by a set of appraisal points to be considered in evaluating external evidence from a study of treatment, a study of diagnosis, or a meta-analysis or systematic review. The appraisal points reflect a number of key influences on the validity and importance of evidence that should be considered in deciding whether it should affect one's current clinical practice. Responses to appraisal points can take a variety of forms ranging from simple binary choices (e.g., pass–fail, yes–no, 1–0; Sackett et al., 2000; Straus, Richardson, Glasziou, & Haynes, 2005) to more graded responses via additional symbols or words (e.g., Pass+, Poor-Minimal-Adequate-Excellent). As we will see, some of the appraisal criteria are easier to rate objectively than others, so additional notes may also be needed. In any event, ratings are to be based on information that is presented in, or can be calculated from, the report of the study. If the information needed for an appraisal point cannot be found or calculated, the evidence must be rated as failing to meet that criterion, although appending the designation UR (unable to rate) might be useful for distinguishing criteria that are failed on this basis from criteria failed for other reasons.

The general idea of critical appraisal is that evidence from studies that meet the appraisal criteria should have a greater impact on clinical practice than evidence whose validity and importance are in doubt. However, it is rare for a study to either pass or fail all of the appraisal criteria; most studies occupy a large middle ground with strengths on some of the criteria and weaknesses on others. It does not appear that ratings across the various criteria can be integrated into a single overall quality rating in any meaningful fashion (e.g., Glasziou, Vandenbroucke, & Chalmers, 2004), although emerging efforts to study the impact of specific criteria on evidence quality (e.g., Simmerman & Swanson, 2001) might eventually make this more feasible. Thus, the critical appraisal process does not guarantee unanimity among evaluators of external evidence, but it does serve three important purposes. First, it enables competent, ethical, and intellectually honest evaluators to make explicit judgments about whether the external evidence suggests that a change in clinical practice should be considered. Second, critical appraisal facilitates reasoned discussions among individuals having different viewpoints about evidence, making it possible to pinpoint specific areas of disagreement. Finally, critical appraisal provides clear direction to researchers concerning the ways in which future studies should be designed to maximize validity and importance of findings.

The final section of the three external evidence critical appraisal forms requires a subjective judgment concerning the validity and importance of the evidence from the study, as a prelude to deciding the clinical bottom line. As defined by Sackett et al. (2000), the clinical bottom line is the clinical action that follows from the paper; here we will define it as a statement about whether the external evidence warrants considering a change to current clinical practice.

Next we consider the specifics of appraising external evidence concerning treatment.

CATE: CRITICAL APPRAISAL OF TREATMENT EVIDENCE

To begin, it is important to specify what is meant by treatment evidence. The terms *treatment, intervention, remediation,* and *therapy* will be used interchangeably to refer to any action undertaken in an effort to improve a client's circumstances with respect to a previously diagnosed communication disorder. This definition is intended to encompass any and all efforts to modify any factor that is believed to be relevant to the patient's current or anticipated communication difficulties and includes anatomical, physiological, cognitive, emotional, behavioral, social, and environmental objectives. Treatment can be aimed at increasing capabilities and/or participation or at decreasing deficits and/or restrictions. Efforts to increase the interpretability of a patient's communicative acts; to improve a client's ability to discriminate words in noise; to enable a patient to use compensatory memory strategies; to reduce the odds that a child will develop a reading disability, as well as efforts to change a client's communication environment, are all encompassed by this definition of treatment.

Figure 6.1 shows the one-page CATE form. It begins with spaces for listing the four components of the FQ addressed by the study, but note that a single study may provide evidence on more than one FQ—for example, a study may report evidence on more than one outcome measure, on more than two treatment conditions, or on more than one kind of patient or problem. When this happens, a separate CATE should be completed for each different FQ because the critical appraisal results are likely to vary according to the question that was investigated.

For example, examine the brief description of Study 1 in Table 6.2 to identify the FQs this study addressed. As you see, evidence is provided on three different outcome measures, and they did not all yield the same results. Even if all of the measures had shown significant differences in favor of the preschool program group, the individual measures might have differed with respect to validity and reliability, blinding, and so forth. Addressing each outcome with a separate CATE form would make it much easier to appraise the evidence concerning that outcome measure and thus to draw conclusions about which, if any, of the results should have an impact on current practice.

By contrast with studies that provide evidence relevant to several FQs, for some studies it is impossible to identify even one complete FQ. This does not necessarily mean that their evidence is not worth appraising, but I would suggest that if two or more PICO components are not specified in a study, it is doubtful that its evidence could meaningfully reduce the uncertainty that motivated the search for external evidence. For example, imagine a school-based SLP who currently uses a pull-out model of service delivery. She and her

---

CATE: Critical Appraisal of Treatment Evidence

Evaluator: Date:

Evidence source:

Foreground question addressed by the evidence:

For	(Patient/problem)
is	(Treatment/condition)
associated with	(Outcome)
as compared with	(Contrasting treatment/condition)

Appraisal points

1. Was there a plausible rationale for the study?
2. Was the evidence from an experimental study?
3. Was there a control group or condition?
4. Was randomization used to create the contrasting conditions?
5. Were methods and participants specified prospectively?
6. Were patients representative and/or recognizable at beginning and end?
7. Was treatment described clearly and implemented as intended?
8. Was the measure valid and reliable, in principle and as employed?
9. Was the outcome (at a minimum) evaluated with blinding?
10. What nuisance variable(s) could have seriously distorted the findings?
11. Was the finding statistically significant?
12. If the finding was not statistically significant, was statistical power adequate?
13. Was the finding important (ES, social validity, maintenance)?
14. Was the finding precise?
15. Was there a substantial cost-benefit advantage?

Validity: Compelling _____   Suggestive _____   Equivocal _____

Importance: Compelling _____   Suggestive _____   Equivocal _____

Clinical bottom line:

Figure 6.1.   A form to guide critical appraisal of treatment evidence (CATE).

supervisor are satisfied with her students' progress, but she attends a workshop that makes her honestly uncertain about whether the collaborative–consultative model of service delivery would have a more favorable cost–benefit ratio. She writes an FQ and conducts a search for external evidence; Study 6 (Table 6.2) is the most relevant study that she finds.

The description of Study 6 suggests two FQs, neither one of which is completely specified due to the absence of a comparison condition. Because there is no contrast and the outcomes of the collaborative–consultative model appear similar to the outcomes that the SLP experiences with her current approach, it seems unlikely that the external evidence from this study would be sufficient to impel her to consider changing to the collaborative–consultative model. For this reason, a full-fledged critical appraisal of the evidence from the study would not be necessary.

Table 6.2. Brief descriptions of six imaginary treatment studies

Study	Description
1	Fourth-grade reading scores were compared in children who had or had not attended a district-sponsored phonological processing program when they were preschoolers, as indicated by a retrospective review of program files. Results showed significantly higher scores on a test of oral reading speed and a test of nonword reading for the group who had attended the pre-school program, but average reading quotients of the two groups did not differ.
2	Five adults with mental retardation were taught to ask for clarification of ambiguous messages using a multiple baseline design. The percentage of ambiguous messages that were verbally queried was recorded daily during a one-week baseline (pre-treatment) phase, after which one participant was selected at random each week to enter a two-week treatment phase. For two participants, clarification requests increased from 0% to 80% after three treatment sessions; no increases were seen in the others.
3	Scores on a test of speech perception were examined in 4-year-old children who had received a unilateral cochlear implant within the previous year. Results showed significantly increased speech perception scores in all participants.
4	High school physical education teachers were invited to attend an educational session on strategies for avoiding vocal abuse that was offered in September. At the end of the school year, teachers completed a survey asking them to estimate the number of school days they missed due to laryngitis. Teachers who attended the educational session reported significantly more laryngitis than teachers who did not attend the session.
5	Pure tone averages and word recognition scores were calculated for adolescents with severe bilateral congenital sensorineural hearing loss when using a hearing aid with frequency transposition and when using a hearing aid without frequency transposition. The order in which the hearing aids were worn for testing was determined randomly for each participant.
6	The use of a collaborative–consultative model of service delivery for speech and language therapy in elementary schools was investigated. Improvements in most students' speech and language skills were observed over the course of the school year, and SLPs, teachers, administrators, and parents were satisfied with results.

Appraisal Points

When one or more clear, relevant, and reasonably complete FQs can be identified, the next step is to evaluate the evidence with respect to the individual CATE appraisal points that are discussed in turn next.

1. Was there a plausible rationale for the study?

As noted earlier, plausible rationales need not only come from theory; clinical observations and clinical experience can and do provide a strong basis for empirical studies. The intent of this criterion is merely to ensure that there is a rationale for the study that goes beyond idle curiosity, chicanery, or greed. Despite the brevity of their descriptions, all of the studies in Table 6.2 have defensible rationales.

2. Was the evidence from an experimental study?

In an experimental study, treatment is actively manipulated for the purposes of the investigation; that is, in an experimental study the treatment is altered in some way such that it differs from what at least some of the participants would have received otherwise. In an observational study, patients receive treatment just as they would have had there been no investigation, although their performance may be recorded and/or described more systematically or in greater detail than usual. As noted in Chapter 4, with all else being equal we can have more confidence in the internal validity of evidence from experimental studies than from observational studies. However, recall that observational studies may sometimes provide the best evidence possible, for example when disorders are extremely rare, when treatment effects emerge very slowly, or when ethical considerations prevent experimental manipulation due to incontrovertible evidence of treatment benefits or harms.

Study 2 and Study 5 in Table 6.2 clearly meet the criterion of involving experimental manipulation. In Study 2 the order in which the participants were treated and the length of time they spent in the pretreatment phase were controlled by the investigator; similarly, in Study 5 the investigator decided when and how the two amplification conditions would occur. Study 4 is difficult to judge based on the information provided, but it would pass this appraisal point if the educational session were only offered because of the study. The remaining studies would not meet this criterion; there is no indication that decisions about which children would attend the preschool phonological processing program were controlled for Study 1, nor was cochlear implantation or the collaborative-consultative model manipulated for the purposes of Study 3 or Study 6, respectively.

3. Was there a control group or condition?

Regardless of whether the study was experimental or observational, it is important to ask whether there was a comparison—of outcomes from different treatment protocols or different treatment phases. The comparison condition need not have been constructed by the investigator—he or she could simply record and compare outcomes from different treatment programs or facilities, for example, but the validity of such uncontrolled comparisons is inherently weak due to the potential for confounding.

A few terminological distinctions concerning comparison conditions might be helpful here. When participants are identified and assigned to different treatment groups in such a way as to minimize their pretreatment differences, the comparison is between parallel groups. When participants are simply followed over the course of treatment in an effort to explore associations between their preexisting characteristics and treatment responses, they are known as a cohort. When participants are selected for a study because they are known to differ on one or more characteristics before they undergo treatment, the study involves a comparison between cases and controls. And in N-of-1 studies, the comparison is between treatment phases in an individual patient rather than between treatment groups: Performance levels may be compared during a pretreatment or baseline phase, an active treatment phase, a posttreatment phase, and a maintenance or follow-up phase.

Of the studies in Table 6.2, four would meet the criterion of having a control group or condition. In Study 1, the comparison is between scores from children who attended the preschool phonological processing program and scores from children who did not. In Study 2, the comparison is between percentages of ambiguous messages queried verbally during the pretreatment phase and the treatment phase for each adult. In Study 4, the comparison is between teachers who attended the educational session and teachers who did not. And in Study 5 the comparison is between the two types of hearing aids. In Study 3 and Study 6, on the other hand, there is no mention of a contrasting condition—the same treatment was provided to all of the participants.

4. Was randomization used to create the contrasting conditions?

As noted in Chapter 4, randomization is the best way to reduce the potential for pretreatment differences to account for the observed treatment effects. Thus, when patients are randomly assigned to differing treatments, or when the order in which patients or goals are selected for treatment is determined randomly in N-of-1 studies, the results are given greater weight for E^3BP. Of the studies in Table 6.2, only Study 2 and Study 5 made use of randomization in constructing the comparison conditions.

5. Were methods and participants specified prospectively?

Prospective studies are valued for two main reasons. First, in prospective studies attempts can be made to recruit participants who are representative of the population(s) of interest and to minimize a priori differences between participants in the contrasting treatment groups. Second, clinicians, examiners, and other study personnel can be trained and monitored to ensure that testing and treatment protocols are being administered as intended.

Study 1 illustrates why evidence from retrospective studies is usually so much weaker than evidence from studies with prospective designs. Despite having a plausible rationale and a control condition, this study's retrospective design makes it unlikely that the investigator will have access to information on the specifics of the phonological processing program, its schedule, its duration and intensity, the characteristics of the people who administered it, or the extent to which it was administered as intended. In addition, because the investigator used preexisting data and had no control over which children received the intervention program and which did not, there is a great risk that the two groups of children differed systematically in other respects before the program began and that any group differences in their fourth-grade reading scores were due to these factors rather than to the program. For example, if the children who attended the program were more likely to have highly educated parents than the children who did not attend it, then differences in the reading scores of the two groups might have resulted not from the program but rather from this sociodemographic factor or a host of other possible influences on their reading scores (the elementary schools they attended, their cognitive skills, their teachers, and so forth). For these reasons, results from retrospective studies must always be interpreted with caution.

6. Were patients representative and/or recognizable at the beginning and the end?

Ideally, the evidence report would provide information on the procedures by which potential participants were identified as well as on the inclusion and exclusion criteria that were imposed. In addition, descriptive information concerning the numbers and characteristics of potential participants who declined or were excluded from the study, as well as of the participants who did and did not complete it, is very helpful in evaluating whether the participants were representative of the target population or demonstrably similar to the patients of interest to the evidence appraiser. Investigators cannot address every conceivable variable of interest, but the information should be adequate to enable readers to judge whether the evidence would apply to the kinds of patients they see.

In addition to information on the participants who began the study, it is necessary to have information on participation attrition, or loss. Attrition is a concern because of the possibility that participants who completed the study were systematically different (in severity, age, intelligence, expectations, motivation, and so forth) from those who did not. If attrition is high (>20%) or if it does not occur approximately equally in the various treatment groups, both the internal and external validity of the findings can be questioned. An analysis showing that participants lost to attrition were similar in major respects to those who completed the study can help to allay these concerns.

When the evidence comes from a randomized controlled trial, a related issue concerns participants who are assigned to one treatment but select an alternative treatment during the course of the study. According to the intention-to-treat (or intent-to-treat) principle, participants should be analyzed according to their original group assignment, even if they opted for a different treatment before the study ended. The intent-to-treat criterion might seem counter-intuitive, but its logic rests on the assumption that once groups have been created by random assignment, anything that alters the original randomization could introduce confounders that threaten the validity of the group comparison. The phrase "Once randomized, always analyzed" reflects the intention-to-treat idea.

None of the brief descriptions of the studies in Table 6.2 provide information that would be needed to pass this appraisal point, and several of the studies seem vulnerable to serious distortions based on the ways in which participants were identified and enrolled. For example, the results of Study 4 showed that teachers who attended the vocal abuse session reported more laryngitis than teachers who did not attend, a finding that could be interpreted as showing that the education session had the opposite of its intended effect. However, if the teachers who attended the session did so because they were more susceptible to laryngitis in the first place, then they would have had more laryngitis than non-attendees regardless of the education session, so the relationship between the session and the outcome cannot be determined.

7. Was treatment described clearly and implemented as intended?

Several issues need to be considered here. Evidence is not useful unless the various treatment conditions are described in enough detail that an experienced clinician can understand their differences and similarities and can envision applying them (perhaps after a period of training). Explicit information (within the page limits of the publication outlet) is needed concerning the treatment procedures; treatment duration and intensity; and the credentials, qualifications, and training of those who provided the treatment. In addition to the idealized descriptions of treatments, evidence that each treatment was implemented as intended (sometimes known as *treatment fidelity*) during the study also increases confidence in the internal validity of the findings. For example, raters blinded to information about the study hypotheses could be trained to rate the occurrence of the distinctive features of a treatment from a randomly selected set of video- or audiotapes to ensure that the features are present at the desired levels over time and across clinicians and patients.

8. Was the measure valid and reliable, in principle and as employed?

This CATE appraisal point concerns the quality of the measures used to document the effects of treatment; concerns about the measures used to identify participants should be addressed under appraisal point 6. As mentioned before, when evidence is provided from more than one measure it is recommended that each measure be addressed on a separate CATE form. Of interest are 1) the measure's validity and reliability in principle for the measurement task and 2) the measure's validity and reliability as actually employed during the study. For example, the validity and reliability of results from a norm-referenced test as reported in the test manual can only be generalized to situations comparable to the norming study, which usually means that each participant took the test only one time. If such a test were administered to the same participant more than once, especially over a relatively short interval, the validity and reliability of its results would be unknown, so measuring change with an alternate form of the test might yield more credible evidence.

Zhang and Tomblin (2003) pointed out another measurement issue that poses a validity threat to pre-post comparisons on norm-referenced tests. Specifically, when low scores on a highly reliable measure are used to qualify participants for a study, the statistical phenomenon of regression to the mean makes it impossible to attribute subsequent improvements on the same measure to treatment or other variables such as recovery, maturation, and so forth, because it is more likely that the second score will move toward the mean than that it will move even farther from the mean. Tomblin, Zhang, Buckwalter, and O'Brien (2003) suggested that this problem can be avoided by administering both the diagnostic (qualifying) measure and a second performance measure at baseline, and comparing improvements to this unbiased estimator of performance rather than to baseline scores on the diagnostic measure itself. Evidence from a treatment study in which measurement is controlled for regression to the mean would thus be substantially stronger than evidence from studies with poor measures and/or or lack of such controls.

Given the problems with repeated administration of most standardized norm-referenced tests, many treatment studies involve criterion-referenced measures, either extant or designed specifically for a particular investigation. Information on validity and reliability for some criterion-reference measures may be available, but in many cases investigators design their own measures to capture the aspects of performance that the treatment is expected to alter. An investigator could provide some evidence concerning a study-specific measure by showing its association with better-known measures, social validity ratings, and so forth. However, when no such evidence is available, it will be necessary to make a subjective judgment about the face validity of the measure, that is, whether it seems reasonable in light of one's knowledge and experience. Needless to say, judgments about measurement validity are open to considerable debate, and so disagreements about this aspect of critical appraisal will not be uncommon.

Regardless of whether a norm-referenced or criterion-referenced measure is used, its reliability in the study, across different examiners and/or over time, should be reported—for example, by reporting the percentage of agreement between independent ratings.

9. Was the outcome (at a minimum) evaluated with blinding?

To pass this appraisal point, the individual(s) who administered the measures of treatment effects or outcomes should have done so without access to any information that could have revealed which treatment the participants had received. This criterion has to be considered separately for every measure of treatment that a study reports and confidence in the conclusions adjusted accordingly. For example, if testing by blinded examiners shows no treatment effect but unblinded patients or family members report significant improvement, the findings from unbiased observers must be accorded more weight in clinical decision making. The use of secretin, a digestive hormone, as a treatment for autism spectrum disorders provides a case in point. As with many new and seemingly powerful treatments, the earliest evidence concerning the effectiveness of secretin came in the form of testimonials by hopeful parents and practitioners. However, several subsequent studies in which observers (parents as well as professionals) were blinded to children's treatment status (e.g., Coplan, Souders, Mulberg, Belchic, Wray, Jawad, et al., 2003; Unis, Munson, Rogers, Goldson, Osterling, Gabriels, et al., 2002) have shown no benefit of secretin. The controls for subjective bias mean that the evidence from studies with blinded observers is more likely to validly reflect the effects of secretin.

While blinding of examiners is essential, blinding of other study personnel also can increase confidence in the validity of treatment evidence. In randomized trials, ideally neither those responsible for assigning patients to groups nor those responsible for communicating the assignments to patients would have access to information that could alter the original, randomly determined assignment. Another layer of security against subjective bias could be imposed by blinding those responsible for analyzing results—for example, by labeling the data from each treatment with an alias and finalizing statistical conclusions before the treatments are identified.

10. What nuisance variable(s) could have seriously distorted the findings?

Judging this appraisal point requires identifying systematic differences between the treatment conditions (other than the treatments themselves) that could have significantly distorted the findings. It would be rare for a behavioral study to be able to control for all such differences, so the focus here should be only on the ones that could invalidate the conclusions about the effects of treatment. For example, imagine a study of a treatment program designed to increase the number of initiations by children with language deficits. Initiations were quantified in a pretreatment language sample recorded as each child interacted with a clinician, and the same clinician then provided 10 individual treatment sessions to children in the experimental group while children in the control group received no treatment. After the 10th treatment session, language samples were recorded again as children in the treatment group and children in the control group interacted with the clinician, and results showed significantly more initiations by children in the treatment group.

At least one nuisance variable here poses a serious threat to the validity of concluding that the treatment program was effective—namely, the children who were treated were much more familiar with the clinician at the time of the final language sample than were children in the control group, and increased familiarity could reasonably be expected to lead to more initiations. Because this nuisance variable would be expected to have a similar effect on the initiations as would treatment, the validity of concluding that treatment affected initiations is doubtful.

Note that some nuisance variables might be expected to have the opposite effect of treatment, in which case they would not be viewed as seriously compromising results in favor of the conclusion that treatment was effective. However, if no treatment effects were found, such nuisance variables would seriously compromise the conclusion that the treatment was ineffective. In short, for this appraisal point it is important to think specifically about whether the nuisance variable could have distorted the conclusions about either positive or null findings concerning the effects of the treatment.

11. Was the finding statistically significant?

This is a straightforward question about whether the p value of the statistical findings concerning treatment is low enough to provide some confidence that the results would be unlikely if the null hypothesis (of no treatment effect) were true.

12. If the finding was not statistically significant, was statistical power adequate?

This appraisal point is very important when drawing conclusions from treatment comparisons that are not statistically significant, because only when statistical power is adequate (conventionally, 0.80 or more) can one be reasonably confident in a conclusion of no difference. Statistical power, p value, ES, and sample size interact with one another, but generally speaking, if p and ES are held constant, studies with larger samples will have more power than studies with smaller samples. Accordingly, if a small study finds no statistically significant effects of treatment but does not report the power of the statistical test and the minimum ES of interest, the validity of concluding that the treatment was ineffective is doubtful.

On the other hand, when a treatment currently being used is found to be ineffective in a study with adequate statistical power, the external evidence would suggest that abandoning the approach in favor of one with better evidentiary support should be considered. For example, in a large RCT examining the impact of tympanostomy tubes on developmental outcomes in otherwise healthy children with persistent middle-ear effusion (Paradise et al., 2003, 2005, 2007), no differences were found between children who received tubes promptly and children who received them up to 9 months later. Because statistical power was > 0.80 to detect a difference between the groups as small as $0.33\ SD$ with $p < 0.05$, results of this study suggest that the practice of using tubes in children similar to those studied in an effort to avoid later deficits in speech, language, cognitive, psychosocial, auditory processing, attentional, and literacy development should be altered in favor of a more conservative approach to management (Berman, 2007).

13. Was the finding important (effect size, social validity, maintenance)?

Appraising this point requires at a minimum a judgment about whether the magnitude of each treatment effect should be viewed as clinically important. For studies with more than one outcome measure, it may be helpful to consider each measure on a separate sheet, especially if you have to estimate them yourself using the methods described in Chapter 5. If the study provides average scores and SDs from different treatment groups, Cohen's d can be calculated for each pair of treatments to reflect the size of each group difference in SD units. If the evidence comes from a correlational study, R^2 can index the strength (but not the directionality) of the association. Odds ratios (either provided or calculated when possible from individual patient outcomes) can indicate whether the odds of each outcome were substantially different across treatment groups. And for N-of-1 studies, ES measures such as d_1, percentage of increase (or reduction), and percentage of nonoverlapping data points can be used to gauge this aspect of importance of treatment evidence. Remember that small effect sizes may nonetheless be judged to be important if they exceed those found in previous studies of treatment for the condition or if few studies of the treatment have been conducted.

In addition to ES, other information can contribute to a judgment about this appraisal point, including whether treatment effects were maintained over time and whether effects were perceptible by people without special expertise in communication skills.

14. Was the finding precise?

As noted in Chapter 5, it is important to consider precision when deciding whether external evidence should alter clinical practice. A study may report a large and statistically significant difference between treatments, but if the ES is surrounded by a wide confidence interval, then the clinical implications are unclear. Studies should report the confidence interval (CI; conventionally at the 95% or 99% level) for each ES, or at a minimum for the point estimates from

Table 6.3. An illustration of the effect of sample size on precision in two studies comparing mean scores from treatment (t) and control (c) groups

Study	N	M_t	M_c	Difference	95% CI
1	200	103	91	12	8.2, 15.7
2	20	103	91	12	−0.7, 24.7

which ES would be calculated. If CIs are not provided, the size of the study sample and the reliability of the measure in question can provide a rough gauge of precision: Findings from small samples are likely to have wide CIs, particularly if derived from measures whose reliability is unknown.

Table 6.3 illustrates the impact of sample size on precision by contrasting the CIs from two studies identical in every respect except sample size: Study 1 had 100 participants in a treatment group and 100 participants in a control group, and Study 2 had 10 participants in each group. After treatment, the mean scores and standard deviations of the treatment ($M = 103, SD = 13$) and control ($M = 91, SD = 13$) groups on a standardized test were the same for both studies, and this difference of 12 standard score points (representing a Cohen's d of 0.92) was statistically significant ($p < 0.05$) in both studies.

Despite all of these similarities, the increased precision of findings from Study 1 makes its treatment evidence far more important than the findings of Study 2. The 95% CI surrounding the average group difference of 12 points is clearly much narrower for Study 1; if the experiment could be repeated 100 times (sampling from the same population), the group mean difference would be expected to fall between 8.2 and 15.7 points, always in favor of the treatment group, 95 times. Because in Study 2 the true value of the group difference could lie anywhere from a slight (0.7 point) advantage for the control group to an almost 25-point advantage for the treatment group, evidence from this study would have much less impact on a clinician considering whether to alter his or her current treatment approach.

CIs can be constructed around correlations as well. Here again, the larger the sample (i.e., the more pairs of scores), the narrower the CI and the more precise the estimated association among the variables. Using the same data sets from the two hypothetical studies described previously, with Ns of 200 and of 20, yields nonsignificant correlations of $r = 0.06$ and $r = -0.18$, respectively, and in both studies the 95% CI extends across $r = 0$, as is typical for a nonsignificant result. But the 95% CI for the larger study would range from −0.14 to 0.24, whereas the CI for the smaller study would encompass a much wider range of possible r values (−0.73 to 0.51), illustrating the general principle that larger samples yield findings of greater precision than do smaller samples.

15. Was there a substantial cost–benefit advantage?

This appraisal point requires considering whether the benefits of a treatment substantially exceed known or potential harms and further whether the benefits are consistent with costs. At present, few treatment studies in communication disorders have explicitly addressed the relative balance of benefits, costs, and risks, partly because of the clinical bias to assume that most treatment efforts will be beneficial, or at least harmless. However, the strongest possible evidence for use in deciding to alter one's current treatment approach would come from studies in which treatments are compared not only with respect to anticipated benefits but also with respect to anticipated and unanticipated harms and costs. Evidence from studies that provide information sufficient to weigh treatment benefits, costs, and harms (whether to patients, families, practitioners, facilities, or third-party payers) should have a relatively greater impact on a decision to change current practice than evidence from studies that do not address costs and benefits explicitly, and such evidence will also be more persuasive in debates over health care financing.

Ratings of Validity and Importance

Following the appraisal points, the CATE form asks for an integrated impression about the validity and importance of the evidence that was appraised, using one of three descriptors (compelling, suggestive, equivocal) that I would define in the following ways. Compelling evidence is virtually incontrovertible, such that unbiased experts would find little or nothing about it to debate. Suggestive evidence is open to debate on a few points, but on balance unbiased experts would be expected to reach similar conclusion about it. Equivocal evidence can be debated on so many points that unbiased experts might reach opposite conclusions about it. Judgments about validity and importance can be made independently; evidence from the same study could be compelling in terms of validity but only equivocal in terms of importance. There are no rules for deciding when external evidence becomes sufficiently valid and sufficiently important that it should affect current practice, but I would suggest the following guidelines. When both the validity and importance of external evidence are compelling, altering one's current clinical approach must be considered seriously (in conjunction with the other two sources of evidence, of course). When either validity or importance of external evidence is equivocal, no change to current practice need be considered (although a change might be considered based on the patient's progress or preference, of course). And when validity and importance of external evidence are both at least suggestive, different clinicians might well reach different decisions about whether to consider altering current practice.

For example, consider again Study 1 in Table 6.2 in which the average fourth-grade reading scores were compared in children who had or had not attended a phonological processing program when they were preschoolers. If scores were 2 SDs higher for children who had attended the program, the confidence interval was narrow, and the program had little cost and no harms, the importance of the evidence from this study might be viewed as at least suggestive and possibly even compelling. However, the validity of the evidence from this study would have to be viewed as equivocal (due to its retrospective design and the lack of information on participants, procedures, measurement quality, controls for subjective bias, and so forth), so this external evidence alone would not justify a decision to implement the phonological processing program more widely.

The Clinical Bottom Line

The clinical bottom line at the end of the CATE is the place to state simply whether the appraisal of the external evidence does or does not support considering a change in one's current treatment approach—whether to adopt a different approach that is not being used or to stop using a current approach due to evidence that is ineffective or harmful.

A Practice CATE

Imagine a clinician uncertain about the optimal approach for helping adolescents and adults generalize a newly acquired speech production skill to settings outside the clinic. His current approach is to ask such patients to sign a contract

Table 6.4. A description of an imaginary treatment study for use in practicing CATE

Background	Treatment for adult speech production deficits often involves a period of acquisition and practice within a therapy setting, followed by a period in which the client is instructed to practice using the new skill in extra-therapy contexts. The present study examined the effectiveness of a device designed to increase the rate at which clients generalize a new speech production skill to extra-therapy settings.
Methods	Over a 3-month period, all patients in a large facility whose clinicians reported that extra-therapy generalization was their only remaining treatment goal were invited to participate. Twenty participants were randomly assigned to an active treatment condition or to a placebo control condition by means of a sealed envelope containing a randomly assigned number; those with even numbers received the active treatment. The facility's receptionist provided each client with a lightweight wristband corresponding to his or her number. Wristbands (approximate cost: $20) were identical in appearance, but wristbands used by the treatment group emitted a slight, unobtrusive tactile sensation once hourly on a varying schedule while wristbands used by the control group were inert. A research assistant unaware of the study's hypotheses or group assignments told participants that the wristbands were intended to help them remember to use their target skill outside of the therapy context and that they were to wear the wristbands between the hours of 9 A.M. and 9 P.M. for the next 5 days, during which time no other treatment was provided. Productions of the target skill during a 10-minute conversation with an unfamiliar research assistant were recorded on the day before clients received the wristband and on the day after the conclusion of the 5-day treatment period. At the end of the study, trained listeners blinded to group assignment counted the number of target skills produced in the randomly ordered samples from each participant. The percentage of agreement between pairs of raters who independently tallied eight randomly selected audiotapes ranged from 89% to 97%.
Results	At baseline, the target skill was produced by the treatment group an average of 2 times $(SD = 1.4)$ and by the control group an average of 3 times $(SD = 1.7)$. In the final sample, the target was produced an average of 5 times $(SD = 1.8)$ by the treatment group and 4 times $(SD = 1.8)$ by the control group $(p < 0.05)$.

CATE: Critical Appraisal of Treatment Evidence

Evaluator: Dollaghan   Date: October 2006

Evidence source: Table 6.4

Foreground question addressed by the evidence:

For adults needing to generalize a speech skill	(Patient/problem)
is a wristband that issues tactile reminders	(Treatment/condition)
associated with increased use of the skill	(Outcome)
as compared with an inert wristband	(Contrasting treatment/condition)

Appraisal points

1. Was there a plausible rationale for the study? — Y
2. Was the evidence from an experimental study? — Y
3. Was there a control group or condition? — Y
4. Was randomization used to create the contrasting conditions? — Y
5. Were methods and participants specified prospectively? — Y
6. Were patients representative and/or recognizable at beginning and end? — N
7. Was treatment described clearly and implemented as intended? — N
8. Was the measure valid and reliable, in principle and as employed? — Y
9. Was the outcome (at a minimum) evaluated with blinding? — Y
10. What nuisance variable(s) could have seriously distorted the findings? — UR
11. Was the finding statistically significant? — Y
12. If the finding was not statistically significant, was statistical power adequate? — NA
13. Was the finding important (ES, social validity, maintenance)? — Y−
14. Was the finding precise? — N
15. Was there a substantial cost–benefit advantage? — UR

Validity: Compelling _____   Suggestive __X__   Equivocal _____

Importance: Compelling _____   Suggestive _____   Equivocal __X__

Clinical bottom line: No need to consider changing current practice.

Figure 6.2.   A sample CATE completed for the evidence from the treatment study described in Table 6.4. (Key: Y = the evidence appears to meet this criterion; Y− = the evidence meets this criterion in some but not all respects; N = the evidence does not meet this criterion; UR = unable to rate this criterion with information provided; NA = not applicable.)

committing them to practice the new skill at least three times a day and in three different settings and to bring notes about these experiences to the following treatment session. Although most of his patients agree to comply with this strategy, he wonders if there is any external evidence showing a better way to speed up the process of extra-therapy generalization. Based on a literature search, the study summarized in Table 6.4 represents best current external evidence. Use the CATE form to rate each appraisal point and to make a judgment about validity and importance before writing the clinical bottom line.

My CATE for the wristband study appears in Figure 6.2. As you see, I think that this study fares well with respect to many factors that could threaten the internal validity of its results. Participants were referred and enrolled consecutively (i.e., they were not hand picked by the investigator or study personnel), and the procedures for randomizing them to groups and assessing the effects of the treatment were also strong due to the blinding tactics that were used. As illustrated by my CATE, I rated this study less highly with respect to several other features of the participants and procedures simply because the summary does not provide any information about the types of patients who were enrolled, about their equivalence pretreatment on features other than their productions of the target skill, or about the specific procedures by which clinicians instructed clients to use the wristbands. The information given makes it difficult to determine whether any nuisance variables might have distorted the results. It seems reasonable to conclude that simple frequency counts were valid measures, and it appears that they were used reliably. The difference in favor of the active wristband group was unlikely to have resulted from random chance, as shown by the statistically significant p value.

The study fared somewhat less well with respect to the importance of its findings. An ES calculated from the prepost difference scores of the two groups suggests that the active group produced about three more target productions in 10 minutes at the end of the study than at the beginning, as compared with an increase of about one production in the placebo group, for an estimated d of about an SD. However, the precision of the findings is not reported, and because the sample size is small, it is likely that the CI would be quite wide. Thus, it is difficult to estimate the true impact of the active wristband on patient performance; the effect could have been quite a bit smaller or quite a bit larger than what was observed in the study. It is also difficult to judge the cost–benefit ratio for the treatment. The wristbands were reasonably inexpensive but no estimate of the cost of the usual treatment for such patients is provided, nor do we know whether clients maintained their increased rates of target production after the study ended. I concluded that the validity of the evidence from this study is suggestive but that its importance is only equivocal. Accordingly, my clinical bottom line is that there is no need for the clinician to consider changing his or her usual approach to treatment with patients, although the clinician might certainly find the results intriguing enough to consider trying something like the placebo wristband approach for individual patients who are not making adequate progress in generalizing their skills outside the therapy room.

SUMMARY

This chapter concerned a set of criteria for deciding whether external evidence suggests that one treatment approach is substantially superior to another. If so, a clinician not using the approach better supported by external evidence would need to consider altering current clinical practice to incorporate it. As will be discussed in Chapter 9, evidence internal to clinical practice and evidence on patient preferences must also be considered in deciding whether a change is warranted. However, a clear understanding of the validity and importance of external evidence concerning a new treatment approach is the first step toward E^3BP.

7

Appraising Diagnostic Evidence

To the extent that clinical economy depends on getting the right treatment to the right people, clinicians are, no matter what their philosophical bent or political point of view, categorizers.

— E.J.S. Sonuga-Barke, 1998, p. 117

Before a client can be treated, he or she must be identified as having the potential to benefit from intervention, or diagnosed. The diagnostic process is essentially one of categorization. We seek to classify people accurately with respect to 1) whether they should be evaluated further (the purpose of screening), 2) whether a disorder or impairment is evident (the purpose of diagnosis), or 3) whether a particular kind of disorder or impairment is evident (the purpose of differential diagnosis). Classification errors are costly. They can prevent people who could benefit from treatment from receiving it in a timely fashion, or from receiving the optimal treatment for their disorder. They can also result in needless anxiety and squandered resources when treatment is recommended for people who do not have a disorder (e.g., Tluczek, Koscik, Farrell, & Rock, 2005). Interestingly, the underlying reason for classifying is the same as the underlying reason for treating—to improve patient outcomes by providing optimal care (Moons & Grobbee, 2002). Critical appraisal of a classification tool (whether for screening, diagnosis, or differential diagnosis) enables a clinician to determine whether the external evidence suggests that a change to a different diagnostic tool should be considered.

Classification is only one of the reasons why we may evaluate, assess, or appraise patients. We also examine communication and related skills after we have diagnosed patients in order to plan and monitor their subsequent intervention. However, because these kinds of assessments are conducted not to classify patients but to improve treatment outcomes, external evidence concerning their value would logically come from studies comparing treatment results from patients with whom they have and have not been used (see e.g., Knottnerus & van Weel, 2002). For example, an investigator could compare acquisition of language forms in children who had randomly been assigned to one of two groups—one in which treatment goals were selected on the basis of a language sample analysis and one in which treatment goals were selected on the basis of elicited imitation. If all children then underwent identical treatment procedures and results were significantly better in one of the groups, that evaluation procedure could be viewed as the better choice for treatment planning. Although this study concerns evaluation procedures, the CATE form described in Chapter 6 would be used to appraise this evidence because it is the impact of the evaluation tools on treatment outcomes, not their classification accuracy, that is of interest in this case.

This chapter, by contrast, focuses on critical appraisal of evaluation tools that are specifically designed to classify people *prior* to making decisions about treatment. Battaglia, Bucher, Egger, Grossenbacher, Minder, and Pewsner (2002) noted that the information needed for these classification decisions can be simple or complex; it can come from elaborate laboratory tests or from answers to a few simple questions during a case history interview. The term *diagnostic* will be used to refer to any such classification procedure, whether it is conducted for purposes of screening, diagnosis, or differential diagnosis. The critical appraisal format is known as CADE: Critical Appraisal of Diagnostic Evidence. As was the case with the CATE, the CADE form was developed by synthesizing criteria and questions from several sources, including Battaglia et al. (2002); Bossuyt et al. (2003); Sackett, Haynes, Guyatt, & Tugwell (1991); Sackett, Straus, Richardson, Rosenberg, & Haynes (2000); the Scottish Intercollegiate Guidelines Network (2001); and Whiting, Rutjes, Reitsma, Bossuyt, & Kleijnen (2003).

The CADE and CATE forms are similar in many respects, but before describing the CADE in detail it is worth highlighting two important differences. First, by contrast with studies of treatment in which participants can be assigned to receive a particular treatment, it is impossible (or at least unethical) to manipulate participants' diagnostic status—people cannot be assigned to have or not to have a disorder in order to examine the accuracy of a diagnostic procedure. Instead, they must be studied as they are when they enter the study. For this reason, diagnostic evidence is not appraised with respect to whether it was obtained in an experimental and/or randomized study. Second, in appraising evidence on a diagnostic measure we will not use effect size metrics but rather metrics that reflect the measure's accuracy in classifying individuals who have, or do not have, the condition of interest.

CADE: CRITICAL APPRAISAL OF DIAGNOSTIC EVIDENCE

To begin, a reminder that the term *diagnostic* will be used to refer to any measure or procedure by which individuals are classified for clinical purposes, so the CADE can be used to critically appraise evidence concerning screening, diagnosis, and differential diagnosis. The CADE does not apply to assessment or evaluation procedures when they are not being used for one of these three classification purposes.

Figure 7.1 shows the CADE form, which begins with spaces for the components of the foreground question (FQ) addressed by the study. For diagnostic evidence, the first (P) component of the foreground concerns identifying a type of patient or problem, and the outcome (O) component always concerns classification accuracy. In addition, for diagnostic evidence the critical comparison is not between two treatment conditions but rather between an *index*

CADE: Critical Appraisal of Diagnostic Evidence

Evaluator: Date:

Evidence source:

Foreground question addressed by the evidence:

    For identifying   (Patient/problem)

    what is the   (Outcome – accuracy)

    of   (Index measure)

    as compared with   (Reference standard)

Appraisal points

1. Was there a plausible rationale for the study?
2. Was the index measure compared to a reference standard?
3. Was the reference standard valid, reliable, and/or reasonable?
4. Were measures and procedures described clearly?
5. Were measures administered independently?
6. Were measures administered with blinding?
7. Were methods and participants specified prospectively?
8. Were participants recognizable and representative of the actual diagnostic task?
9. Were the reference standard and the index test both administered to all participants?
10. Was LR+ (sensitivity/1 – specificity) $\geq$ 10.0?
11. Was LR– (1 – sensitivity/specificity) $\leq$ 0.10?
12. Was precision adequate?
13. Was there a substantial cost–benefit advantage?

Validity: Compelling ___   Suggestive ___   Equivocal ___

Importance: Compelling ___   Suggestive ___   Equivocal ___

Clinical bottom line:

Figure 7.1. A form to guide critical appraisal of diagnostic evidence (CADE).

measure (the diagnostic procedure being evaluated) and what is known as a *reference standard* (or *gold standard*), defined as the "best available method for establishing presence or absence of the target condition" (Bossuyt et al., 2003, p. 8).

The reference standard could consist of a combination of diagnostic indicators or measures; single definitive or pathognomonic markers are rare even in medicine. In addition, the reference standard does not have to be infallible—there are very few perfectly accurate diagnostic tools, even for well-known and much-studied diseases (Faraone & Tsuang, 1994). Even if there is no widely agreed gold standard for a disorder, some means of distinguishing affected from unaffected individuals must be specified and defended. For example, expert clinicians' judgments about the presence or absence of the target disorder could provide the best available "tin" reference standard in the early stages of investigation of a poorly understood disorder such as childhood apraxia of speech or auditory processing disorder (Dollaghan, 2003). Finding that such judgments can be made consistently would be a first step toward specifying the particular characteristics that underlie them, a necessary precursor not only to clinical progress but also to theoretical understanding. To quote Bailey (1994, p. 15): "Theory cannot explain much if it is based on an inadequate system of classification." In short, a reference standard is critically important to the quality of diagnostic evidence.

As was the case with the CATE form, if a single study provides evidence on more than one FQ—for example, it involves more than one index measure or reference standard—separate CADEs should be completed so that findings concerning each comparison can be evaluated individually.

Appraisal Points

If one or more reasonably complete FQs can be identified, the diagnostic evidence can be appraised with respect to each of the following appraisal points. As noted in Chapter 6, some of the points can be answered with a relatively simple and objective binary (Yes–No) judgment whereas others rely more heavily on subjective judgment. When this is the case, making a brief note about the reason for the rating is helpful in understanding disagreements with other appraisers.

1. Was there a plausible rationale for the study?

A passing score on this appraisal point merely requires a reasonable rationale for studying the index measure, whether based on theory, previous research, or clinical observation.

2. Was the index measure compared with a reference standard?

The only way to evaluate the accuracy of an index measure is by directly comparing its findings to those of the reference standard; neither group mean comparison studies nor correlational studies provide much more than a plausible rationale for future studies of a measure's accuracy. For example, the fact that there is a difference between the mean score of a group of cases (people who have the disorder) and the mean score of a group of controls (people who do not have the disorder) on a new diagnostic measure does not allow inferences about the accuracy with which the measure would assign each individual to the correct group. Similarly, the fact that scores on a new measure correlate significantly with scores on an existing measure does not allow inferences about the new measure's accuracy in classifying individuals as cases or controls. Even if such studies seem to suggest that a new measure is worth examining more closely, they cannot yield evidence that is nearly as credible or important as studies in which the classification decisions of the index measure are compared directly to those of a reference standard.

3. Was the reference standard valid, reliable, and/or reasonable?

Evaluating the quality of the reference standard can be difficult when there is no universally accepted method for diagnosing the condition. When the reference standard is a norm-referenced test, a number of criteria for psychometric adequacy have been described (e.g., McCauley, 2001; McCauley & Swisher, 1984), but these are neither necessary nor sufficient to guarantee the test's diagnostic accuracy. When no information on the validity or reliability of the reference standard is available, it should at least appear reasonable for the diagnostic task (Sackett, Haynes, Guyatt, & Tugwell, 1991), an impression that probably depends on a combination of the measure's face validity and tradition (i.e., whether it has been used for diagnosis in the past). Several investigators have pointed out the need for additional attention to the quality of gold standards themselves as new methods emerge for evaluating the validity of diagnostic markers (e.g., Demissie, White, Joseph, & Ernst, 1998; Johnson, Gastwirth, & Pearson, 2001) and the diagnostic category distinctions they are intended to capture (e.g., Dollaghan, 2004b; Lenzenwenger, 2004; Meehl, 2004; Ruscio & Ruscio, 2004). However, in the meantime, the answer to this third appraisal point depends on subjective judgments about the reference standard that are open to debate.

4. Were the index measure, reference standard, and testing procedures described clearly?

The reference standard and the index measure both need to be described clearly enough that an experienced clinician can understand their differences and similarities and can envision applying them (perhaps after a period of training). In addition, information on the qualifications, training, and reliability of those responsible for administering the measures and on the specific procedures employed in the study is needed to enable the rater to identify any significant variables that could have distorted the findings.

5. Were the index measure and the reference standard administered independently?

6. Were the index measure and the reference standard administered with blinding?

Appraisal points 5 and 6 should be easy to answer with a simple "yes" or "no." They concern the potential for subjective knowledge or expectations to influence results of either the reference standard test or the index test—a phenomenon known as clinical review bias (Battaglia et al., 2002). As noted earlier, subjective bias is very difficult to avoid even for measurement tasks that seem to be simple and objective; many measures of communication disorders require subjective and/or perceptual ratings that are susceptible to the influence of inadvertent biases even when examiners are skilled and conscientious. For this reason, evidence on the diagnostic accuracy of the index test is more likely to be valid when the potential for subjective bias is controlled, first by ensuring that the index and reference measure are not administered by the same examiner, and second by ensuring that examiners have no information about the participant(s) that could systematically influence the way in which they administer, score, or interpret the results. Ideally, examiners would be assigned at random to administer either the reference standard or the index test to a participant about whom they have no other information. Additional tactics (e.g., blinding of other study personnel including statisticians) would likewise contribute to the internal validity of the resulting diagnostic evidence.

7. Were methods and participants specified prospectively?

As was the case for treatment evidence, prospective studies of diagnostic accuracy have a number of advantages. Prospective recruitment and enrollment of participants offers the potential for better control over selection bias or unrecognized nuisance variables that could systematically distort the representativeness of the study sample. Prospective studies also enable important methodological controls, such as independent, blinded test administration, tests of inter-examiner reliability, and checks on the fidelity of test procedures to be imposed.

8. Were participants recognizably representative of the actual diagnostic task?

This appraisal point concerns the crucial question of whether the index measure's classification accuracy was assessed in a sample of participants who are recognizable and representative of the actual diagnostic task. Of interest here are the total number of participants and the percentage of participants who had (were positive for) the diagnostic condition of interest according to the reference standard, which is known as the *base rate* of the disorder in the sample. It is a good idea to get into the habit of estimating the base rate in any study of a diagnostic tool because variations in base rate across different samples can lead to substantially different estimates of accuracy for some commonly reported accuracy metrics (though not the two that are recommended here). Information on how many participants failed to complete one or both of the diagnostic measures and the reasons for this attrition should be examined because the accuracy of the index measure could be inflated if it were calculated only for some of the participants.

In addition to sample size, base rate, and attrition, information on the participants should be examined with respect to some specific biases that can threaten the validity of evidence from a diagnostic study. One, spectrum bias, can occur if the accuracy of the index measure is studied only in preselected or hand-picked cases and controls, whose diagnostic status (positive or negative) is obvious. The problem here is analogous to the problems introduced when patients are not assigned randomly to groups in studies of treatment. Namely, myriad confounders could affect the kinds of patients who do and who do not get selected for the study, making it impossible to know whether the results concerning the accuracy of the diagnostic measure would apply to a more representative group that included individuals whose diagnostic status was less clear cut (Battaglia et al., 2002; Sackett et al., 2000). The threat of spectrum bias is one reason why diagnostic measures that have been found accurate in a variety of clinical facilities are valued more highly than measures that have been tested in a more restricted range of clinical settings and participants.

9. **Were the reference standard and the index test both administered to all participants?**

Differential verification bias (or verification bias) can occur if the diagnostic status of some, but not all, of the participants in a sample is determined ("verified") by direct testing with the reference standard. This problem applies equally when participants are presumed to be free of the target disorder based on absence of previous clinical concern or service and when participants are presumed to have the target disorder based on a previous diagnosis with some other measure. In either case, the assumption that their performance on the reference standard can be predicted is unwarranted. Unless the diagnostic status of all of the participants in a diagnostic study is determined in an identical fashion, using the study's reference standard, the accuracy of the index measure cannot be determined with confidence. Accordingly, diagnostic evidence is stronger if all participants, regardless of diagnostic group, are administered both the reference standard and the index test.

10. **Was LR+ [sensitivity/(1 – specificity)] ≥ 10.0?**

11. **Was LR– [(1 – sensitivity)/specificity] ≤ 0.10?**

Appraisal points 10 and 11 on the CADE concern likelihood ratios, the preferred metrics for examining the extent to which the index test provides important diagnostic information, accurately distinguishing those individuals who are affected by the target disorder from those who are not with reference to the best available diagnostic measure. Although true diagnostic status is a complex construct and approaching it as a dichotomy has been criticized (e.g., Feinstein, 2002), virtually all of the literature concerning diagnostic evidence focuses on classifying people as affected or unaffected. This means that there are two distinct types of accuracy that need to be considered in evaluating a diagnostic measure—its success in identifying those who have the disorder and its success in identifying those who do not. A variety of measures of diagnostic accuracy exist, including sensitivity, specificity, positive predictive value, negative predictive value, positive and negative likelihood ratios (LR+ and LR–), diagnostic odds ratio (e.g., Glas, Lijmer, Prins, Bonsel, & Bossuyt, 2003), and the area under the Receiver Operating Curve (ROC). The LR+ and LR– are the two metrics that are preferred currently (Battaglia et al., 2002; Bossuyt et al., 2003). Likelihood ratios can be calculated from the precursor metrics of accuracy known as *sensitivity* and *specificity* (Battaglia et al., 2002) that are easy to determine from a four-fold, or 2x2, table.

2x2 Tables for Diagnostic Evidence   The 2x2 table format for examining evidence on the accuracy of a diagnostic measure can be seen in Table 7.1. Each of the four cells in the table itself is labeled with a letter (*a–d*). The caption at the top of the table defines two columns labeled with plus (+) and minus (–) signs. The column headed with a plus (+) sign locates participants who are positive (+) for the target disorder according to the reference (gold) standard. It might help to think of this entire group of participants as the "Haves" because, according to their performance on the reference standard, they have the disorder. The column headed with a minus (–) sign is for the people who are negative (–) for the target disorder according to the reference standard. You can think of these participants as the "Have-Nots" in the sample that was studied. The total number of people with the disorder appears outside the table, at the bottom of the left-hand column, and the total number of people without the disorder appears outside the table, at the bottom of the right-hand column. As you look for evidence of a measure's diagnostic accuracy, you want to remember that the sum of cells *a* and *c* must equal the total number of Haves in a study. The sum of cells *b* and *d* must equal the total number of Have-Nots. The sum of the Haves and the Have-Nots will be the total number of participants in the study, and the percentage of Haves out of the total number of participants is the base rate (or prevalence) of the disorder in the study's sample.

The rows of the table are also labeled with plus (+) and minus (–) signs. In this case, however, the + and – signs refer to diagnostic status according to the results of the index test rather than according to the gold standard. You will not need to worry about the sums of the rows right now, but you can see that the sum of cells *a* and *b* represents the total number of people that the index (new) test identifies as having the disorder. The sum of cells *c* and *d* represents the total number of people that the index test identifies as not having the disorder.

Now that you see what is happening outside the table, in its margins, consider what actually goes inside the table in cells *a* through *d*. The left-hand column represents all of the people who have the disorder according to the reference standard. Some of these people will also be diagnosed as Haves by the index measure. These are known as the true positive cases, and they belong in cell *a* because they are identified as having the disorder (+) by both the reference and the index measure. The remaining Haves in the left-hand column are those whom the new measure classifies, incorrectly, as not having the disorder. These false negative cases belong in cell *c*. Again, cells *a* and *c* must sum

Table 7.1.   Diagnostic 2x2 table

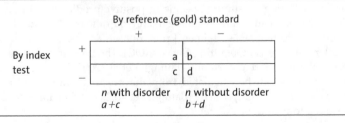

to the total number of people diagnosed as having the disorder according to the reference standard.

Cells *b* and *d*, or the right-hand column of the table, are reserved for people diagnosed by the gold standard as not having the disorder. The index test will correctly identify some of these people as not having the disorder. These true negatives belong in cell *d* because they score in the negative (–) range on both measures. Cell *b* will then contain the remaining Have-Nots whom the new test incorrectly identifies as having the disorder. These cases are known as false positives. Table 7.2 shows the descriptive labels for cells a, b, c, and d.

Consider the following information as it might be presented in a study of a new diagnostic measure:

One hundred children previously diagnosed with language impairments (LI) according to state standards and 100 children with normal-range scores according to state standards (LN) were administered the Perfect Expressive Receptive Measure (PERM), a new diagnostic test. Eighty of the children with LI and 30 of the children with LN scored in the language-impaired range on the PERM.

These two sentences contain all the information you need to set up a complete 2x2 table. Begin by drawing and labeling a 2x2 table, and be sure to put the true diagnostic status (positive [+] or negative [–] for the target disorder) according to the reference test at the top of the left and right columns, respectively. To the left of the table, indicate diagnostic status according to the index test, which in this case is the PERM. Label the top row positive (+) and the lower row negative (–).

The next step is to figure out the total number of people diagnosed with the disorder according to the reference standard (the Haves; in this case, those with LI) and the number without the disorder according to the reference standard (the Have-Nots; in this case, those with LN). What was the reference standard in this investigation? Although we do not know the details, state standards were applied to identify 100 children with LI (the Haves) and 100 children with LN (the Have-Nots). Where do these numbers go? Remember that they reflect the total number of people diagnosed with and without the disorder by the reference standard.

If you put 100 at the bottom of each column, outside the table proper, then you are exactly right. Now it is time to think about the numbers that actually

Table 7.2. 2x2 table with cells labeled

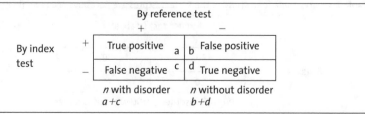

go inside the table in cells *a* through *d*. Eighty of the 100 children with LI, according to the gold standard, scored in the language-impaired (i.e., +) range on the PERM, so the number 80 goes in cell *a*.

What about cell *c*? Cells *a* and *c* have to add up to 100, and 80 children were assigned to cell *a*. Therefore, the number 20 must go in cell *c*, reflecting the number of children with LI who scored in the normal (–) range on the PERM.

Thirty of the 100 children with LN scored in the language-impaired (+) range on the PERM, so this number goes in cell *b*. That leaves 70 children who scored in the non–LI range on both the reference standard and the PERM, so 70 is the number that goes in cell *d*. Your 2x2 table should look like the one in Table 7.3.

This example involved one kind of diagnostic task—separating individuals who have a disorder from those who do not. The same logic and 2x2 table format are involved in studies of screening and studies of differential diagnosis. In a study of screening, for example, the reference standard is the best available screening test for distinguishing individuals who should be evaluated further (+) from those whose performance does not warrant clinical concern (–). In a study of differential diagnosis, all of the participants will have previously been diagnosed with a disorder; in this case, the reference measure is the best available method for distinguishing individuals who have a certain type or subcategory of the disorder from those who do not.

For example, use the following brief description of an imaginary study to construct another 2x2 table:

> *Of 312 patients with speech production disorders, genetic abnormalities were found in 31, 22 of whom also had abnormal performance on the new auditory pitch perception test. Seventy-three of those who had normal genetic findings had abnormal performance on the auditory pitch perception test.*

This example is included to illustrate that even information that seems confusing at first glance can be deciphered to construct the 2x2 table. First, it is important to recognize that this is not a study of a measure designed to separate people with speech disorders from people with normal speech. Instead, this study concerns the accuracy of a new pitch perception test for distinguishing between those people whose speech disorders are accompanied by genetic abnormalities and those people who have speech disorders but normal genetic findings. This is a problem of differential diagnosis, but fortunately the steps in

Table 7.3. 2x2 table for a study of the Perfect Expressive Receptive Measure (PERM)

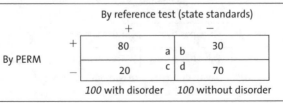

		By reference test (state standards)	
		+	−
By PERM	+	80 a	b 30
	−	20 c	d 70
		100 with disorder	*100* without disorder

setting up the 2x2 table are always the same. Based on the description, we know that the total number of participants in the study was 312. We also can see that the reference standard to be placed at the top of the 2x2 table is the genetic test, with its findings of abnormal (+) or normal (–). According to the description, 31 people had abnormal genetic findings, so 31 goes at the bottom of the left-hand column, outside the margin of the table. None of the remaining people in the original sample of 312 had abnormal genetic findings, so the number of people negative for genetic findings is 312 – 31= 281. This number goes at the bottom of the right-hand column, again outside the table margin. The base rate of genetic abnormalities in this study (i.e., the percentage of people with abnormal genetic findings out of the total number assessed) was 31/312 or 9.9%.

Now it is possible to figure out what numbers belong in cells *a* through *d*. Start with the left-hand column. Cell *a* contains the 22 people whose performance on the new pitch perception test was abnormal (and thus consistent with the findings of the genetic test). Cell *c* contains the remaining nine people required for the column to sum to 31; these nine people had genetic abnormalities but normal pitch perception.

The wording of the information concerning those with normal genetic findings by the reference standard was intentionally designed to be confusing: *Seventy-three of those without genetic abnormalities had abnormal pitch perception.* The sentence reveals that 73 people with normal (negative) genetic findings had abnormal (positive) pitch perception, and so this number belongs in cell *b* (the conjunction of normal genetic and abnormal pitch perception results). Subtracting 73 from the total number of people in this column (281) leaves 208, the number that belongs in cell *d*. Table 7.4 shows the completed 2x2 table for this study.

Sensitivity and Specificity   With a 2x2 table, it is simple to understand and calculate two values that are prerequisites to determining the accuracy of the index measures: its sensitivity and its specificity. These terms are often confused, so it is helpful to remember that each one of them concerns just one of the categories defined by the gold standard. Sensitivity concerns only those people who have (are positive for) the disorder, and specificity concerns only those people who do not have (are negative for) the disorder. In explaining or calculating each one, it is helpful to always start by saying which group is involved. To calculate sensitivity, the question should be phrased as follows: *Of*

Table 7.4.   A 2x2 table for an imaginary study of a new pitch perception test

| | | Genetic findings | | |
		+		–
Pitch perception test results	+	22	a b	73
	–	9	c d	208
		31		281

the people who have the disorder according to the reference standard, what proportion does the new test identify as having the disorder? To calculate specificity, the question is: *Of the people who do not have the disorder according to the reference standard,* what proportion does the new test identify as not having the disorder? Phrasing the questions this way makes it clear that calculating sensitivity involves only the left-hand column in the 2x2 table (cells *a* and *c*) because that column contains all the people positive (+) for the disorder according to the gold standard. Sensitivity is simply the proportion of people who have the target condition according to the reference standard (i.e., the sum of cell *a* and cell *c*) who are correctly identified by the new measure (i.e., the number of people in cell *a*). In short, sensitivity = $a \, / \, a + c$.

Specificity concerns only the people in the right-hand column, all of whom are negative (–) for the disorder according to the reference standard. Specificity is the proportion of all the people in this column (i.e., the number in cell *b* plus the number in cell *d*) who are identified as negative (–) by the new test (i.e., those in cell *d*). Thus, specificity = $d \, / \, b + d$.

The sensitivity and specificity of the PERM can be calculated from Table 7.3. The sensitivity of the PERM for identifying children with language impairments according to state standards is $a \, / \, a + c$ (i.e., 80/100 or 0.80). The specificity of the PERM for identifying children who have normal language according to state standards is $d \, / \, b + d$ (i.e., 70/100 = 0.70). From Table 7.4, we can determine that the sensitivity of the pitch perception test for identifying people whose speech disorders are accompanied by genetic abnormalities is in people with speech production disorders is $a \, / \, a + c$ (i.e., 22/31, or 0.71). The specificity of the pitch perception test for identifying people who have speech disorders but normal genetic findings is $d \, / \, b + d$ (i.e., 208/281, or 0.74).

Positive and Negative Likelihood Ratios Sensitivity and specificity have largely been supplanted by two accuracy metrics known as positive and negative likelihood ratios (abbreviated as LR+ and LR–, respectively). There are several reasons for this change, including the susceptibility of sensitivity and specificity to variations in the base rate of the sample in which they are studied. Bossuyt et al. pointed out that any measure of diagnostic accuracy reflects "the behavior of a test under particular circumstances" (2003, p. 9), and with a little thought you can see how a measure's classification accuracy would be likely to differ according to the severity levels of affected participants in the sample, the extent to which the sample contains participants whose disorders are easily confusable with the diagnostic condition of interest, and so forth. This is one reason why it is so important to avoid selection, spectrum, and differential verification bias in seeking strong diagnostic evidence. Sensitivity and specificity are also highly susceptible to variations in the base rate of the diagnostic condition in the sample from which they are derived. As you recall, the base rate of the target condition in a sample is the percentage of people who have the disorder out of the entire sample of people who were assessed (i.e., affected and unaffected people). If the base rate in the sample is 50% (i.e., the ratio of affected to unaffected people is about 1:1, or half the people have the condition and half do not), then prior to administering the diagnostic test, the probability that any individual has the disorder is 50%. However, as the base rate in a sample decreases, there are by definition relatively fewer people with the disorder and relatively more who are unaffected by it. In such a sample, specificity will automatically be higher than in a sample with a 50% base rate because there is a higher probability that the correct diagnosis is "normal" before the diagnostic measure is even administered. Conversely, sensitivity will automatically be lower in a sample with a low base rate than in a sample with a 50% base rate because there are fewer affected people to identify, so the probability that the correct diagnosis is "disordered" is lower before the test is given.

The susceptibility of sensitivity and specificity to base rate variations limits their usefulness as accuracy metrics, especially when they are derived from samples in which the base rate is low. This is not uncommon in the behavioral sciences, where many studies of diagnostic tests involve samples with base rates of 10% or lower. It is important to realize that in such a sample, a specificity of .90 for the index test is far from impressive—simply guessing that every member of the sample is "normal" would also be correct 90% of the time. Similarly, sensitivity is likely to be lower than specificity in samples with low base rates, regardless of the quality of the diagnostic measure being studied.

Likelihood ratios are not impervious to sample characteristics, but they are substantially less affected by base rate than are sensitivity and specificity (Sackett, Haynes, Guyatt, & Tugwell, 1991), primarily because likelihood ratios are derived from sensitivity and specificity considered simultaneously. As noted by many authors, when the base rate of a sample is 50%, sensitivity, specificity, and LR+ and LR– will all lead to the same conclusions about the accuracy of a diagnostic measure. However, when the base rate is extremely low or extremely high, likelihood ratios are preferred.

Roughly speaking, the LR+ reflects confidence that a positive (disordered or affected) score on a test came from a person who has the disorder rather than from a person who does not. The formula for calculating the LR+ is sensitivity/(1 – specificity). You can see that this boils down to the ratio of the test's accuracy in identifying true positive cases (sensitivity) to its false positive rate (1 – specificity). The LR+ for a level of test performance in the affected range, then, provides an index of the confidence we can have that a person who obtains a positive (affected or disordered) score on the test truly (i.e., according to the gold standard) does have the disorder. Thus, the higher the LR+ for a positive score on the test, the greater the confidence that a person who obtains a positive score has the disorder.

If LR+ indicates confidence that a score in the affected range comes from an affected rather than an unaffected person, you can probably guess that the LR– concerns confidence that a score in the unaffected range comes from a person who truly does not have the target disorder. The formula for the LR– for a score in the unaffected (negative, normal) range on the index test is (1 – sensitivity)/specificity, or the ratio of the measure's false negative rate (1 – sensitivity) to its true negative rate (specificity). The lower the LR– for a diagnostic measure, the greater the confidence that a person who obtains a normal-range score does not have the disorder.

Likelihood ratios can extend from 0 to infinity, and because they reflect probability scales it is not possible to define a nonarbitrary value at which an LR+ becomes sufficiently high, or LR– becomes sufficiently low, to ensure the importance of a diagnostic result. If the likelihood ratio (either positive or negative) for a given test result is 1.0, the finding has no diagnostic value—it is just as likely to have come from a person with the disorder as from someone who is unaffected by the disorder. Beyond that, however, various authors have used varying verbal descriptors to characterize LRs, usually in terms of how much the test result changes our view of the likelihood that the patient has the disorder (Ebell, 1998; Sackett, Haynes, Guyatt, & Tugwell, 1991). Sackett, Straus, Richardson, Rosenberg, & Haynes (2000, p. 72) noted that "diagnostic tests that produce big changes from pretest to posttest probabilities are important and likely to be useful to us in our practice"; Table 7.5 summarizes some values and descriptors of LR+ and LR– adapted from Sackett et al. (1991, 2000). As you see, when the pretest probability of the disorder is at least 33%, a positive (abnormal) score on a measure with a LR+ of 10 or more increases the probability to 83%, often allowing a conclusive diagnosis that the patient has the disorder (Ebell, 1998). On a measure with an even higher LR+, a positive score can be interpreted even more confidently as indicating that the patient has the disorder; Sackett et al. (1991, p. 128) noted that for diagnosing alcohol dependency or abuse, answering "yes" to three of four questions has an LR+ of 250. On the other hand, findings with positive LRs below 10 are less informative; LRs in the range of 3–4 are described as merely suggestive that the patient has the disorder.

At the other end of the scale, for classifying patients as free of the disorder, when a patient obtains a normal-range score on a measure with an LR– at or

Table 7.5. Values and descriptors for positive and negative likelihood ratios (LR+ and LR–)

Positive likelihood ratio (LR+)			Negative likelihood ratio (LR–)		
Value	Descriptor	Interpretation	Value	Descriptor	Interpretation
≥ 10	Very positive	Positive (abnormal-range) test score very likely to have come from person with the disorder (post-test probability ≥ 83% for pre-test probabilities ≥ 33%)	≤ 0.10	Extremely negative	Negative (normal-range) test score very unlikely to have come from person with the disorder (post-test probability ≤ 5% for pre-test probabilities ≤ 33%)
3	Moderately positive	Positive test score suggestive but insufficient to diagnose disorder	≤ 0.30	Moderately negative	Negative test score suggestive but insufficient to rule out disorder
1	Neutral	Positive test score uninformative for diagnosing disorder	1	Neutral	Negative test score uninformative for ruling out disorder

Sources: Sackett, Haynes, Guyatt, & Tugwell (1991) and Sackett, Straus, Richardson, Rosenberg, & Haynes (2000).

below 0.10, the presence of the disorder is effectively ruled out. When a measure has an LR– even closer to zero, such as 0.05 or 0.01, then we can be even more confident that a person who obtains a negative (normal range) score on the test does not have the disorder in question. And negative LRs around 0.30 are again suggestive but insufficient to rule out the disorder.

It seems clear that a measure with an LR+ of 2 has inadequate accuracy for diagnosing a person with a disorder, but a decision about whether to use diagnostic measures with LR+s in the neighborhood of 3–4, or even 5–9, depends on one's tolerance for failing to identify affected individuals. Similarly, diagnostic measures with LR– values in the neighborhood of 0.30 could be defended if the consequences of misdiagnosing someone as having a disorder are not serious—but it is very difficult to imagine that the consequences are ever trivial for such classification errors. Perhaps the best thing that can be said about intermediate-range likelihood ratios is that they might lead to further studies aimed at refining the diagnostic measures or to studies aimed at determining whether stronger evidence of accuracy can be found in studies in which diagnostic measures are combined.

The foregoing description of LR+ and LR– is a slight oversimplification that does not address the specifics of how to estimate the pretest probability of the disorder for a particular patient and then to convert it to the posttest probability using the LR for the diagnostic result. A number of authors have suggested using a visual shortcut known as a nomogram for this purpose (Sackett et al., 1991, 2000). To read a likelihood ratio nomogram (see Figure 7.2; see also Sackett et al., 1991), begin by using whatever evidence you can gather to estimate the pretest probability that the patient has the disorder in question. In most cases, this will reduce to the prevalence of the disorder, although the probability of the disorder could be much higher if the patient is being assessed in a facility that specializes in assessing and treating the disorder. Line a straight edge up with the pretest probability so that it passes through the LR+. It will lead to the posttest probability that a person who obtains a positive score on the test has the disorder. For example, if the disorder has a pretest probability of 20% and the test has a LR+ of 20, then the probability is nearly 90% that a person who obtains a positive score on the test has the disorder. For a pretest probability of 10% and an LR+ of 20, the probability of the disorder with a positive test score is slightly more than 70%. You will see by experimenting with the nomogram that as LR+s become larger, so do the probabilities that people who score in the affected range have the disorder.

The same logic and procedures show how LRs interact with pretest probability to allow an estimate of the probability that a person who obtains a negative (unaffected) score has the disorder. For example, with a pretest probability of 20% and a LR– of 0.20, the probability is less than 5% that a patient with a negative score has the disorder. This posttest probability drops to 2% when the LR– is 0.10.

Using a nomogram is a good way to get comfortable with the relationship between likelihood ratios, pretest probabilities, and posttest probabilities. However, prevalence information is not readily available for many behavioral disorders. In addition, many diagnosticians do not remember to carry a nomo-

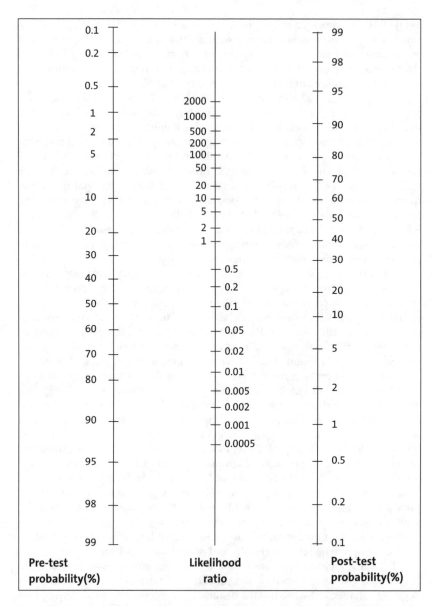

Figure 7.2. Nomogram for converting pre-test probabilities to post-test probabilities for a diagnostic test result with a given likelihood ratio. (Reprinted by permission from Center for Evidence-Based Medicine, Institute of Health Sciences, Oxford, United Kingdom; http://www.cebm.net/likelihood_ratios.asp.)

gram with them at all times. McGee (2002) suggested that for the vast majority of clinical applications in which pretest probabilities of the disorder range between 10% and 90%, likelihood ratios can be interpreted independent of specific pretest probabilities with minimal error.

The best way to get a feel for likelihood ratios is to calculate and interpret some. Start with the PERM, which you calculated to have sensitivity of 0.80 and specificity of 0.70. Here are the resulting LR+ and LR–:

LR+ = sensitivity/(1 – specificity)

     = 0.80/(1 – 0.70)

     = 0.80/0.30

     = 2.67

LR– = (1 – sensitivity)/specificity

     = (1 – 0.80)/0.70

     = 0.20/0.70

     = 0.29

Looking back at Table 7.3, what do these likelihood ratios reveal about the diagnostic usefulness of a positive (affected) and a negative (unaffected) score on the PERM? The LR+ suggests that a score in the "language-impaired" range on the PERM is not very helpful because such a score is only marginally more likely to come from a person with a language disorder than from a person with normally developing language. Similarly, a normal-range score on the PERM is somewhat suggestive of normal language skills, but this conclusion could not be drawn with confidence without further testing.

What would happen to the likelihood ratios if we kept the specificity of the PERM as 0.70 but increased its sensitivity to 0.90 rather than 0.80? Take a minute to make a prediction: Do you expect LR+ to change? If so, in which direction? Now calculate the new likelihood ratio.

LR+ = sensitivity/(1 – specificity)

     = 0.90/(1 – 0.70)

     = 0.90/0.30

     = 3.0

Well, LR+ improved, at least a little. But even when sensitivity seems to be high, the resulting LR+ does not even reach the intermediate level, suggesting again that the PERM's accuracy for diagnosing affected people is inadequate. Even if we bump sensitivity up to a near perfect 0.99, the LR+ remains less than 4.0.

LR+ = 0.99/(1 – 0.70)

     = 0.99/0.30

     = 3.3

These higher sensitivity values have a much bigger impact on LR– , as shown below if specificity remains at 0.70 but sensitivity is 0.90 or 0.99:

With sensitivity $= 0.90$

With sensitivity $= 0.99$

LR– $=$ (1 – sensitivity)/specificity
  $=$ (1 – 0.90)/0.70
  $=$ 0.10/0.70
  $=$ 0.14

LR– $=$ (1 – sensitivity)/specificity
  $=$ (1 – 0.99)/0.70
  $=$ 0.01/0.70
  $=$ 0.01

Are you surprised that improving sensitivity has a far larger effect on ruling out disorder than on ruling in the disorder? If so, you are not alone, but here is the reason. If we have a measure that is perfectly sensitive to the disorder, meaning that it identifies every person who has the disorder, then someone who scores in the normal range must be free of the disorder.

What if we change the PERM's original specificity rather than its sensitivity? You can probably anticipate what will happen, although it may still seem counter-intuitive at first. Keep the PERM's original sensitivity (0.80) and figure out the LR+ for specificity levels of 0.90 and 0.99:

With specificity $= 0.90$

With specificity $= 0.99$

LR+ $=$ sensitivity/(1 – specificity)
  $=$ 0.80/(1 – 0.90)
  $=$ 0.80/0.10
  $=$ 8

LR+ $=$ sensitivity/(1 – specificity)
  $=$ 0.80/(1 – 0.99)
  $=$ 0.80/0.01
  $=$ 80

As you see, improving the specificity of a diagnostic measure greatly increases the likelihood that someone who scores in the disordered range really has the disorder. The logic here, again, is that because a measure with perfect specificity will never mistakenly classify an unaffected person as having the disorder, someone who scores in the disordered range must really have the disorder.

However, what happens to LR– if we increase specificity to 0.90 and 0.99 while maintaining the original sensitivity (0.80)? (Remember that the original specificity of 0.70 resulted in an LR– of 0.29.) The answer, as shown below, is "not much":

With specificity $= 0.90$

With specificity $= 0.99$

LR– $=$ (1 – sensitivity)/specificity
  $=$ (1 – 0.80)/0.90
  $=$ 0.20/0.90
  $=$ 0.22

LR– $=$ (1 – sensitivity)/specificity
  $=$ (1 – 0.80)/0.99
  $=$ 0.20/0.99
  $=$ 0.20

As shown below, even if sensitivity and specificity are both 0.90, the resulting likelihood ratios do not attain the target levels of 10 and 0.10—a fact that should give diagnosticians pause when external evidence reports describe measures with values of 0.90 (or lower) in glowing terms.

LR+ $=$ sensitivity/(1 – specificity)
  $=$ 0.90/(1 – 0.90)
  $=$ 0.90/0.10
  $=$ 9

LR– $=$ (1 – sensitivity)/specificity
  $=$ (1 – 0.90)/0.90
  $=$ 0.10/0.90
  $=$ 0.11

In fact, it is only when both sensitivity and specificity are greater than 0.90 that likelihood ratios at compelling levels are attained, as illustrated next for a case in which sensitivity and specificity are both 0.99:

$$LR+ = [sensitivity/(1 - specificity)] \quad LR- = [(1 - sensitivity)/specificity]$$
$$= 0.99/(1 - 0.99) \qquad\qquad = (1 - 0.99)/0.99$$
$$= 0.99/0.01 \qquad\qquad\qquad = 0.01/0.99$$
$$= 99 \qquad\qquad\qquad\qquad = 0.01$$

Table 7.6 shows positive and negative likelihood ratios for varying values of sensitivity and specificity.

To make sure that you understand how to calculate and interpret LR+ and LR-, examine the 2x2 table concerning the accuracy of the auditory pitch perception test for classifying people whose speech production disorders were and were not accompanied by genetic abnormalities (Table 7.4). The sensitivity of the pitch perception test in this study was 0.71 (22/31) and the specificity was 0.74 (208/281). The resulting LR+ is 2.73, so an abnormal score on the pitch perception test would not be helpful as an indicator of a genetic abnormality. Similarly, because the LR- is 0.39, a normal score on the pitch perception test would not be helpful in identifying people who don't have a genetic abnormality.

12. Was precision adequate?

The previous section showed that likelihood ratios are less vulnerable to sample characteristics than are sensitivity and specificity, but LRs derived from any given sample are point estimates and as such it is important to consider not only their values but also their associated confidence intervals (CIs). The CI, again, indicates range of possible values around an observed value (here, LR+ and LR-) within which its true value can be expected to fall with a known probability. If the likelihood ratios for an index measure are precise (i.e., their surrounding 95% CIs are narrow), that measure is more important for diagnostic decision making than measures that yield less precise information.

Appendix 1 in Sackett et al. (2000) contains an overview and formulas for determining CIs for studies of diagnosis and screening. Another source for this information is Appendix 2 in Battaglia et al., 2002 (available at http://www.ispm.unibe.ch/files/file/261.Bayes_library_handbook.pdf). However, any of several free programs, such as the statistical calculator in the EBM Toolbox at http://www.cebm.utoronto.ca will accept numbers in the 2x2 table

Table 7.6. Examples of the impact of variations in sensitivity (sens) and specificity (spec) on positive (LR+) and negative (LR-) likelihood ratios

Sensitivity	Specificity	LR+ [sens/(1 – spec)]	LR- [(1 – sens)/spec]
0.50	0.50	1.00	1.00
0.60	0.60	1.50	0.67
0.70	0.70	2.33	0.43
0.80	0.80	2.67	0.29
0.90	0.90	9.00	0.11
0.99	0.99	99.00	0.01

format and calculate sensitivity, specificity, likelihood ratios, and associated CIs for an index test, making it easy to determine the precision of the LR values.

If the external evidence being appraised does not provide the frequencies needed to construct the 2x2 table, sample size might be considered in appraising the likely precision of the accuracy metrics. All else being equal, values derived from larger samples will be more reliable than measures derived from smaller samples, with smaller standard errors and narrower CIs. Table 7.7 illustrates this point by comparing the 95% CIs from two studies identical with respect to base rate, sensitivity, specificity, LR+, and LR−, but having different sample sizes (N of 200 and N of 20, respectively). As you see, CIs around each likelihood ratio are considerably wider for the study with the smaller sample. If the sample size is small, it must be assumed that CIs would be wide and the diagnostic tool would yield imprecise results.

Another important feature of CIs that is especially relevant for small sample studies of diagnostic measures is that CIs cannot be calculated with confidence unless there is some variation in classification accuracy. Thus, CIs cannot be calculated when either sensitivity or specificity is perfect (1.0 or 100%). When this occurs, most statistical programs will insert a symbol (usually an asterisk) in place of the missing CI values. It is important not to confuse these asterisks, which indicate uncertainty and a lack of evidence on precision, with the asterisks that are used to indicate statistically significant findings. Asterisks appearing in CIs should suggest skepticism about the reported accuracy values, at least until they have been replicated in multiple, carefully conducted, and large-scale studies of a diagnostic measure.

As a clinician choosing a screening/diagnostic test, how much error are you willing/able to tolerate in classifying a patient? Spotting an asterisk or an infinity symbol in a CI suggests that the measure is not adequately precise to be clinically useful, but beyond these extremes there is no absolute cut-off value for adequate precision. One suggestion would be to examine the value at the "worse" end of the CI to see whether that degree of potential inaccuracy in classifying a patient is tolerable. In Table 7.7, for example, the lower bound of the 95% CI for LR+ in the sample with 20 participants is 1.13, which is perilously close to the completely equivocal likelihood ratio value of 1.0. In other words, based on this small sample study, a score in the disordered range on the index measure provides about as much evidence on a participant's true diagnostic status as would flipping a coin. It is unlikely that a clinician contemplating whether to adopt a new index test would be comfortable with this

Table 7.7. Confidence intervals (CIs) for accuracy metrics from two studies, one with 20 participants and one with 200 participants

Accuracy metric	Value	95% CI (N = 20)	95% CI (N = 200)
Sensitivity	0.80	0.44, 0.98	0.71, 0.87
Specificity	0.70	0.35, 0.93	0.60, 0.78
Positive likelihood ratio (LR+)	2.67	1.13, 7.66	1.98, 3.70
Negative likelihood ratio (LR−)	0.29	0.08, 0.87	0.19, 0.42

degree of diagnostic uncertainty.

13. Was there a substantial cost–benefit advantage?

Answering this question requires considering the cost–benefit ratio of the index measure over the reference standard, both with respect to the ratio of benefits over risks or harms and with respect to whether the financial and time requirements of the index measure are consistent with its diagnostic value. For example, a diagnostic tool that imposes health risks such as increased radiation exposure would need to be justified in terms of its accuracy and impact on clinical outcomes. Similarly, there may be little reason to alter current practice to adopt a new measure that has no clear advantages for the clinician, the facility, or the patient. Particularly when resources are limited, different appraisers may reach different conclusions concerning the balance of clinical value, risks, and costs for the index measure being appraised. Note that the CADE form can provide a clear rationale for decisions about whether to adopt not only index measures reported in the scientific literature but commercially produced diagnostic measures based on information in their test manuals.

Ratings of Validity and Importance

Just as was the case with the CATE form, this section of the CADE requires an integrated judgment over the various appraisal criteria about whether the validity and importance of the external evidence were compelling (unarguable), suggestive (debatable on a few points but leading to a consistent conclusion), or equivocal (debatable on so many points that unbiased and competent raters could reach opposite conclusions). If validity and importance are both compelling, there is serious reason to consider adding or adopting the index measure for use in diagnostic decision making. If either validity or importance of external evidence is equivocal, no change to current diagnostic practice needs to be considered (although a change might be considered based on the particular patient's characteristics or preferences, of course). And if validity and importance of external evidence are both at least suggestive, different clinicians might well reach different decisions about whether to consider using the index measure for diagnosing the condition.

The Clinical Bottom Line

The clinical bottom line at the end of the CADE is the place to state simply whether the appraisal of the external evidence does or does not support considering a change in one's current diagnostic approach—whether to adopt a new diagnostic measure or to stop using an inadequate diagnostic measure.

A Practice CADE

Table 7.8 contains a description of an imaginary study. If you were asked to make a recommendation about whether this school district should adopt the new measure rather than the one currently in use, to what conclusion would your CADE of this external evidence lead? To answer this question, the first

Table 7.8. Description of an imaginary diagnostic (screening) study for evaluation with CADE

Background	A new, 10-minute screening measure for identifying preschool children with communication disorders has recently become available. The present study was designed to determine whether the shorter (5-minute) screening measure currently used in a school district should be replaced by the new measure.
Methods	Caregivers of all children presenting for a kindergarten readiness session (N = 2000) in a large school district were invited to participate. Consent forms were obtained for 1,000 children, who were randomly assigned to be screened with either the district's current screening measure or the new measure. For each screening measure, all children who failed it and an equal number of randomly selected children who passed it were administered a diagnostic battery by research assistants unaware of screening results. The diagnostic battery results (positive or negative for presence of communication disorder) were treated as the reference standard.
Results	Seventy children who failed the district's current screening measure and 70 randomly selected children who passed it completed the diagnostic battery. Diagnostic battery results showed communication disorders in 70 children, 50 of whom had failed the district's current screening measure. Diagnostic battery results were negative (no communication disorder) in 70 children, 50 of whom had passed the district's current screening measure. The diagnostic battery was also administered to 100 children who failed the new screening measure and 100 children who passed it. The diagnostic battery showed communication disorders in 115 children, 95 of whom had failed the new screening measure. Diagnostic battery results were negative for 85 children, 80 of whom had passed the new screening measure.

step is to recognize that Table 7.8 provides evidence on two screening measures: the one currently in use and the new one. For each measure, the FQ would read: "For identifying preschoolers in need of further evaluation (for potential communication disorders), what is the accuracy of this screening measure as compared with the results of a diagnostic evaluation?"

A CADE for the new screening measure is shown in Figure 7.3. The validity of the evidence concerning this measure is at least suggestive, as several precautions were taken to protect against subjective bias. In fact, with the exception of a lack of information about the participants, the index measure, and the reference standard (the diagnostic evaluation), this evidence fares well on most of the appraisal points, and the same would be true of the district's current screening measure since the same research procedures were used.

Calculating the likelihood ratios for the two screening measures, however, shows that they differ in accuracy. As compared to the gold standard diagnostic battery, the sensitivity and specificity of the district's current screening measure were both 0.71 (50/70), yielding an LR+ of 2.5 (95% CI, 1.68 to 3.73) and an LR– of 0.40 (95% CI, 0.27 to 0.60). The sensitivity of the new screening measure was 0.83 (95/115) and its specificity was 0.94 (80/85), so the resulting LR+ was 14.04 (95% CI, 5.98 to 33.00) and the LR– was 0.18 (95% CI, 0.12 to 0.28). Accordingly, my CADE for the new screening measure indicates that both its validity and importance are at least suggestive. My CADE for the cur-

---

CADE: Critical Appraisal of Diagnostic Evidence

Evaluator: *Dollaghan*   Date: *October 2006*

Evidence source: *Table 7.8*

Foreground question addressed by the evidence:

For identifying *preschoolers in need of further evaluation*	(Patient/problem)
what is *the accuracy*	(Outcome – accuracy)
of *the new screening test*	(Index measure)
as compared with *results of a diagnostic evaluation*	(Reference standard)

Appraisal points

1. Was there a plausible rationale for the study?   Y
2. Was the index measure compared to a reference standard?   Y
3. Was the reference standard valid, reliable, and/or reasonable?   Y
4. Were measures and procedures described clearly?   N
5. Were measures administered independently?   Y
6. Were measures administered with blinding?   Y
7. Were methods and participants specified prospectively?   Y
8. Were participants recognizable and representative of   Y
   the actual diagnostic task?
9. Were the reference standard and the index test both   Y
   administered to all participants?
10. Was LR+ [sensitivity/(1 – specificity)] $\geq$ 10.0?   Y
11. Was LR– [(1 – sensitivity)/specificity] $\leq$ 0.10?   N
12. Was precision adequate?   Y
13. Was there a substantial cost–benefit advantage?   Y

Validity: Compelling _____   Suggestive __X__   Equivocal _____
Importance: Compelling _____   Suggestive __X__   Equivocal _____

Clinical bottom line: *Consider using the new screening test.*

Figure 7.3. A CADE form completed with the evidence on a new screening measure described in Table 7.8.

rent measure, on the other hand, would suggest that importance was equivocal. As a result, even though the new screening measure requires twice as much time to administer (10 minutes rather than 5), its increased accuracy suggests that it would be a better choice than the district's current screening measure.

SUMMARY

This chapter addressed a process for appraising the validity and importance of external evidence on screening, diagnostic, and differential diagnostic measures. The CADE provides a structured format for deciding whether external evidence strongly supports the use of one such tool over another when the goal is to classify individuals accurately. The CADE also enables people with different opinions about diagnostic measures to specify their points of agreement and disagreement. Finally, appraising diagnostic evidence critically reveals the gaps and flaws that need to be addressed in future studies to increase confidence in the measures by which screening, diagnosis, and differential diagnosis of communication disorders are accomplished.

8

Appraising Systematic Reviews and Meta-Analyses

*Meta-analysis makes
me very happy.*
—Jacob Cohen, 1990, p. 1310

Systematic reviews and meta-analyses synthesize external evidence across multiple studies that have been identified and analyzed according to explicit and transparent procedures. The emphasis on explicitness and transparency differentiates systematic reviews and meta-analyses from traditional literature reviews, in which the author makes subjective decisions about which information to include and to highlight. In a systematic review or a meta-analysis, the goal is to use more objective criteria for including, excluding, and evaluating studies so as to provide a more valid, less biased view of the entire evidence landscape concerning a question.

The main difference between systematic reviews and meta-analyses is that the results of a meta-analysis are presented quantitatively in the form of a summary statistic (and its associated confidence interval [CI]) that averages the findings from individual studies. Most meta-analyses concerning the effects of treatment report an average d statistic, but average correlation coefficients, odds ratios and so on, may also be reported. In general, there have been fewer meta-analyses of diagnostic studies to date (see Deeks, 2001; Tatsioni et al., 2005), but in such studies the summary statistic takes the form of one or more averaged accuracy metrics, such as sensitivity, specificity, and/or likelihood ratios. As mentioned in Chapter 5, a forest plot of findings from the individual studies may be helpful in thinking about the consistency and precision of findings that contributed to the overall summary statistic.

Systematic reviews and especially meta-analyses are prized for a number of reasons. First, they provide tangible indications of the importance of converging evidence by illustrating that the findings of a single study are rarely conclusive. This is why many external evidence rating systems assign the highest rank to evidence that is supported by not just one but multiple well-conducted meta-analyses, although Glasziou, Vandenbroucke, and Chalmers (2004) recently made a persuasive argument in favor of systematic reviews over meta-analyses. Second, both systematic reviews and meta-analyses may make it possible to see orderly patterns in a seemingly chaotic research literature, by highlighting the ways in which findings may vary systematically according to the samples, designs, procedures, analyses, and quality features of individual investigations. These advantages make it wise to begin a search for external evidence with recent meta-analyses and systematic reviews before proceeding to appraise individual studies. However, as with any form of evidence, meta-analyses and systematic reviews have to be appraised critically with respect to the validity and the importance of their findings.

A form to guide a critical appraisal of a systematic review or a meta-analysis (CASM) is shown in Figure 8.1. Like the CATE and the CADE forms, the CASM has been constructed from suggestions found in a variety of sources

---

CASM: Critical Appraisal of Systematic Review or Meta-Analysis

Evaluator: Date:

Evidence source:

Foreground question addressed by the systematic review or meta-analysis:

For	(Patient/problem)
is	(Treatment/condition)
associated with	(Outcome)
as compared with	(Contrasting treatment/condition)

Appraisal points

1. Was there a comprehensive and clearly described search for relevant studies?
2. Were clear and adequate criteria used to include and exclude studies from analysis?
3. Were individual studies rated independently?
4. Were individual studies rated with blinding?
5. Was inter-rater agreement adequate?
6. Was an average effect size (treatment) or accuracy metric (diagnosis) presented?
7. Were results weighted by sample size?
8. Was the confidence interval adequately precise?
9. Did a forest plot suggest reasonable homogeneity of findings across individual studies?
10. If not, was a heterogeneity or moderator analysis conducted?
11. Were the results sufficiently relevant to my patient and practice?

Validity: Compelling_____   Suggestive_____   Equivocal_____

Importance: Compelling_____   Suggestive_____   Equivocal_____

Clinical bottom line:

Figure 8.1. A form to guide critical appraisal of systematic reviews or meta-analyses (CASM).

including Ebell (1998); Sackett, Haynes, Guyatt, and Tugwell (1991); Sackett, Straus, Richardson, Rosenberg, and Haynes (2000); Straus, Richardson, Glasziou, and Haynes (2005); and the Scottish Intercollegiate Guidelines Network (2001). The CASM skirts several controversial statistical issues specific to the problem of combining findings across studies, and as methods for conducting meta-analyses of findings from observational studies continue to evolve (e.g., Stroup, Berlin, Morton, Olkin, Williamson, Rennie, et al., 2000), the particular appraisal points may need to be expanded. In its present form, however, the CASM highlights some of the main issues to be considered in deciding whether a systematic review or meta-analysis should contribute to a decision to alter a current clinical approach.

CASM: CRITICAL APPRAISAL OF SYSTEMATIC REVIEWS AND META-ANALYSES

The CASM begins with a section for the foreground question (FQ) addressed by the meta-analysis or systematic review. If an FQ is not evident, then the results of the meta-analysis or systematic review will necessarily be less useful for clinical decision-making than if the analysis had been undertaken with a clear goal in mind. Depending on the number and types of studies available in an area, the FQ may be phrased in relatively broader or narrower terms (Robey & Dalebout, 1998), and myriad factors could be used to constrain the FQ, including the characteristics of participants (e.g., age, disorder, time post onset) and the characteristics of the treatment approach (objectives, procedures, intensity, outcome, and so forth). However, at present there are a number of areas of communication disorders in which the pool of investigations is relatively small, so FQs will necessarily be broad. In such cases, meta-analyses and systematic reviews may be more helpful in guiding future research than for deciding whether a change to current clinical practice is warranted.

Appraisal Points

After the FQ has been identified, the CASM form lists 11 questions that can be used in appraising the meta-analysis or systematic review critically. Some of these appraisal points relate specifically to the quantitative findings that are provided in meta-analyses and will not be used in appraising systematic reviews.

1. Was there a comprehensive and clearly described search for relevant studies?

By contrast with individual treatment and diagnostic studies, where it is usually not feasible to include every potential participant in the study sample, the ideal sample for a meta-analysis or systematic review would consist of every well-conducted study of the FQ ever conducted. Unpublished studies are sometimes sought out and included on the assumption that studies with statistically significant findings are more likely to be published than studies with nonsignificant results, a publication bias that could invalidate the results of the analysis. However, the inclusion of unpublished evidence is controversial because factors other than null findings, such as poor methodological quality, also prevent studies from being published. Whether unpublished studies are included, a graph known as a *funnel plot* is sometimes recommended as a way to estimate whether publication bias might have influenced the results in favor of studies with significant findings. In a funnel plot, the *d* values of the studies that were analyzed are plotted against their sample sizes (smaller to larger; see Figure 8.2). If the resulting graph looks like an inverted funnel (i.e., increased similarity among effect sizes reported in the few studies with large samples at the top of the plot, with a fairly symmetrical distribution of findings from individual smaller-sample studies on either side of the average or summary *d* value), then it is reasonable to conclude that studies with null or negative findings were adequately represented. If there are few or no studies on the left side of the funnel, it is reasonable to conclude that the results may be biased in favor of studies finding significant benefits of treatment, suggesting that the meta-analytic results should be viewed with more caution. Although a symmetrical funnel plot cannot guarantee valid results, it can act as a reminder that the validity of a meta-analysis depends on including as much high quality evidence as possible, regardless of whether the evidence refutes or supports the clinical practice in question.

In addition to published and unpublished studies, meta-analysts may consult experts in an area in an effort to identify evidence that would otherwise have been missed, including evidence from studies published in other languages (Egger et al., 1997, as cited in Jueni, Witschi, Bloch, & Egger, 1999). Accordingly, a positive answer to the first question on the CASM requires that the search strategy (databases and other data sources) be described clearly and in sufficient detail to enable the appraiser to judge whether results have been

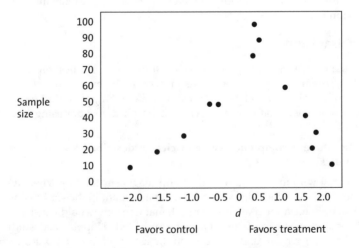

Figure 8.2. Funnel plot of individual studies of treatment. Symmetry suggests no bias against studies with null or negative findings concerning effects of treatment.

derived from a reasonably comprehensive sample of the universe of studies on the FQ.

2. Were clear and adequate criteria used to include and exclude studies from analysis?

This appraisal point concerns the criteria by which studies were judged to be eligible for inclusion in the review or analysis. Because meta-analyses depend on certain statistical information, some of these criteria are straightforward, and studies must be excluded if the necessary information is not reported and cannot be calculated or obtained by contacting a study's author after the fact.

Equally important but much more controversial are criteria for excluding studies based on their design or methodological characteristics. It is not a simple or straightforward matter to assess the quality of the methods used in different studies, at different stages of investigation, and in different topic areas, but most investigators agree that the validity of a systematic review or meta-analysis depends on the validity of the individual studies on which it is based. For example, Jueni et al. (1999) examined 17 meta-analyses of a medical treatment to determine whether results varied according to the methodological quality of the individual clinical trials that were included. They found no consistent effect of methodological quality as rated by 25 different quality rating scales, but when they focused specifically on "the 3 key domains that have been shown to be associated empirically with bias: concealment of treatment allocation, blinding of outcome assessments, and handling of dropouts and withdrawals" (p. 1056), they found that meta-analysis results were significantly more favorable toward treatment when studies in which examiners were not blinded to the treatment group were included. Rather than excluding studies from meta-analyses based on omnibus quality rating scales, these investigators recommended that the relevant methodological features be identified and examined individually, within the context of the current literature in an area, and that the critical influences on bias and confounding always be considered in interpreting meta-analytic results. Similarly, Stroup et al. recommended "using broad inclusion criteria for studies, and then performing analyses relating design features to outcome" (2000, p. 2010), for example, by contrasting the results from studies with and without blinding of examiners or with or without randomization. If it appears that findings differ substantially according to variations in methodological (or other) features, then the meta-analyst might decide not to calculate a single effect size (ES) averaged across all studies (see Westwood, Whiting, & Klejinen, 2005). At the least, any such variations should be described explicitly when the results of the meta-analysis are reported.

3. Were individual studies rated independently?

4. Were individual studies rated with blinding?

5. Was inter-rater agreement adequate?

These three appraisal points concern not the quality of the original studies but the quality of the methods by which information from those studies was coded and summarized for the meta-analysis or systematic review, particularly with respect to the steps taken to reduce threats to its internal validity. Systematic reviews and meta-analyses inherently employ observational designs, so minimizing the potential for subjective bias is crucial. Stronger evidence will come from systematic reviews and meta-analyses in which more than one person independently rated the characteristics, eligibility, and results of individual studies, and for which evidence of adequate inter-rater agreement can be provided. Blinding raters to key information, such as authors and publication dates of studies, is highly desirable although complete concealment may not be possible if all raters have expertise in the content area being analyzed. Including some raters who have no prior knowledge of research studies in the area and documenting high rates of inter-rater agreement are two ways to allay concerns about the possible impact of subjective bias on the coding decisions.

6. Was an average ES (treatment) or accuracy metric (diagnosis) presented?

7. Were results weighted by sample size?

8. Was the confidence interval adequately precise?

The next questions on the CASM form are specific to meta-analyses and concern the importance of the findings. When an average ES or accuracy metric is presented with its CI, and if individual studies were weighted according to sample size so that the average was not unduly influenced by studies with small samples, the reader can judge the magnitude and the precision of the averaged findings more confidently. For example, if the meta-analysis concerns controlled experimental studies of treatment of outcome, then d is the most likely ES metric. For studies with observational designs (including studies of diagnosis), R^2, odds ratios, an ES for a proportions test (Robey & Dalebout, 1998), or a summary receiver operating characteristics curve (Irwig et al., 1994) could be used. Robey and Dalebout provided mathematical equations for calculating various ESs for studies of treatment and pointed out that when ESs are averaged across studies, it is important to weight them "so that effects obtained from small samples (which are more likely to be extreme) are not unduly influential in the calculated value of the average" (1998, p. 1235). They provided a formula for calculating d, the average weighted and corrected ES, from the values of d reported in individual studies. They also described how to calculate its associated 95% CI. When the studies included in the meta-analysis involve large samples and similar findings, the summary statistic will be precise, with a relatively narrow 95% CI. However, when a meta-analysis includes a variety of samples and ESs, then the average ES will be surrounded by a wide CI. Heterogeneous and imprecise findings will necessarily be less helpful to a clinician who is trying to determine whether the weight of the external evidence should motivate a change in his or her clinical practice.

9. Did a forest plot suggest reasonable homogeneity of findings across individual studies?

10. If not, was a heterogeneity or moderator analysis conducted?

The next two questions on the CASM serve as reminders of the need to consider not just the average ES but the consistency of the findings that contributed to it. As described in Chapter 5, in many meta-analyses of treatment studies the average ES is accompanied by a graphic representation of the ESs and precision of the individual studies on which it is based, known as a *forest plot* or *Forrest plot* (Lewis & Clarke, 2001). An example of a forest plot constructed from data presented in a meta-analysis of the effects of treatment on measures of overall phonological development by Law, Garrett, and Nye (2004), appears in Figure 8.3. This figure shows the values of *d* and associated 95% CIs from six individual studies in which overall phonological scores were compared for groups of children who either did or did not receive treatment.

This forest plot contains a great deal of information. For example, we can see that treatment was found to be most beneficial in the study by Almost and Rosenbaum (1998), and that Shelton, Johnson, Ruscello, and Arndt (1978) found that the average score of the control group was higher than that of the treated group following intervention. It is also possible to use the forest plot to identify the studies in which the difference between the treated and untreated group is most likely statistically significant at a low *p* value by recalling that statistically significant findings are most likely when the CI does not cross zero. We can guess that the study by Glogowsa, Roulstone, Enderby, and Peters (2000) probably had the largest sample size, given its narrow CI.

All of these questions could be answered based on the numerical data shown in Figure 8.3 alone—a forest plot is not a mandatory component of a meta-analysis. But being able to look at a picture of the individual studies is helpful in forming an impression of the strength, direction, consistency, and precision of findings from the studies included in the meta-analysis, as well as the relationship of the individual studies to the average or summary value of *d*. Even if a forest plot is not provided, constructing one for yourself by using

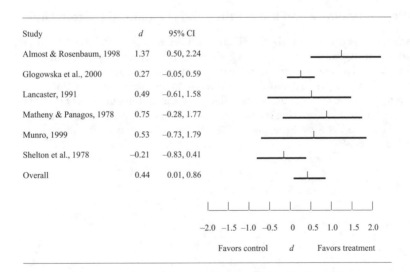

Figure 8.3. Forest plot concerning effects of treatment on measures of overall phonological development constructed with values of *d* and confidence intervals (CI). (Reprinted with permission from The efficacy of treatment for children with developmental speech and language delay/disorder: A meta-analysis by Law, J., Garrett, Z., and Nye, C. *The Journal of Speech, Language, and Hearing Research, 47*[4], 932. Copyright 2004 by the American Speech-Language-Hearing Association. All rights reserved.)

the ESs and CIs reported for the individual studies can help prevent the tendency to oversimplify the state of the literature by assuming that the average ES reflects unanimity of findings across studies.

There is no absolute definition of *reasonable homogeneity* among findings. But if the results of multiple studies, especially those with large samples, are in a consistent direction favoring the treatment in question, then the external evidence would suggest that current clinical practice might need to be altered to incorporate that treatment. When the forest plot shows variable and conflicting findings, a heterogeneity or sensitivity analysis may sometimes be provided in which findings are seen to be more consistent in certain subgroups, such as studies with blinding, patients in a certain age range, and so forth. Such analyses may be suggestive, but their impact on clinical decision making is limited by their retrospective nature, the difficulty of anticipating and analyzing all of the relevant variables, and the reduced number of studies in each subgroup.

11.   Were the results sufficiently relevant to my patient and practice?

The next question on the CASM is a reminder that even if the external evidence from a meta-analysis strongly and consistently favors a particular treatment, it is still necessary to consider whether the patients and treatment protocols that were studied were sufficiently similar to our own patient(s) and practices to inspire confidence that the results would apply. Regardless of how strong the external evidence from a meta-analysis or systematic review may be, it must still be integrated with evidence concerning the characteristics and preferences of a particular patient before a decision about changing current clinical practice is made.

Ratings of Validity and Importance and the Clinical Bottom Line

Finally, as was the case for the CATE and the CADE forms, the CASM includes lines for an overall assessment of whether the validity and the importance of the meta-analysis or systematic review are compelling, suggestive, or merely equivocal, appraisals that should lead directly to the clinical bottom line: How strongly does the external evidence reflected in the systematic review or meta-analysis suggest considering a change in current clinical practice? The answer to this question is a prelude to considering the other two kinds of evidence needed for E³BP.

9

Appraising Patient/ Practice Evidence

> *However robust the research, clinicians face the dilemma of applying this evidence to individual patients.*
>
> —Griffiths, Green, and Tsouroufli (2005, p. 1)

The previous chapters have focused on external evidence from systematic scientific investigation—what we might think of as E^1 of E^3BP. The next two chapters concern E^2 and E^3—evidence from clinical practice and evidence on patient preferences. The fact that this handbook contains a lot more information on external evidence than on the other two kinds simply reflects the current state of the literature, in which specific proposals for obtaining, appraising, and using evidence from clinical practice and evidence on patient preferences have been in relatively short supply. However, interest in these two components of E^3BP appears to be growing, and well-specified methods and rules of evidence concerning E^2 and E^3 seem to represent the next frontiers for E^3BP.

Several of the principles and processes that have been discussed in relation to external evidence can be transferred directly to evidence from clinical practice and evidence on patient preferences. However, there are two major differences that can be discussed with the metaphors of telescopes, microscopes, and white boxes.

TELESCOPES, MICROSCOPES, AND WHITE BOXES

A telescope is an instrument for obtaining information across a broad swath or field, which could range from a city street all the way up to the galaxy or even the universe. In a sense, when we seek, evaluate, and use external evidence from research, we act as telescopes, attempting to capture all of the potentially relevant information in a particular corner of the universe of evidence defined by a foreground question (FQ). The resulting picture is of a broad landscape in which the resolution for examining individual entities is usually poor.

A microscope, on the other hand, is designed specifically to provide a detailed view centered on a particular entity or its component microstructure. When we use a microscope, we can learn a lot about the individual object, but the fine-grained resolution of the instrument prevents us from seeing its relationship to the broader context of other objects. In a sense, when we seek to integrate information obtained from the broad universe of external evidence with evidence from clinical practice with a patient, it is as if we are shifting from a telescope to a microscope. As we zoom in on evidence concerning an individual patient, it is worth remembering that it may sometimes be difficult to reconcile information from the two sources—the criteria for valid and important evidence differ somewhat between the macro and the micro views.

The white box metaphor specifically relates to evidence concerning patient preferences. Here, too, we are zooming in on a particular patient, thus using something more like a microscope than a telescope. However, we cannot directly observe our patient's preferences and values. Unlike evidence from research and evidence from clinical practice with a patient, this information is not accessible to empirical verification by people other than the patient. For this reason, subjective experience has sometimes been characterized as a *black box*, a term that is used in engineering to describe a system whose observable behavior can be predicted even though its internal structure cannot be observed. However, the computer engineering metaphor of a *white box* is even more applicable with respect to obtaining evidence on a patient's preferences. Like a black box, a white box is a system that cannot be observed directly, but at least some of its internal structure is familiar to those who try to understand it. We are akin to white box testers as we use empathy and our own experiences to try to obtain valid and important evidence about the preferences of our patients.

Seeking evidence about the white box of patient preferences is the topic of Chapter 10. This chapter focuses on using something like a microscope to obtain independently verifiable evidence about clinical practice with a particular patient to be integrated with evidence of the other two kinds in clinical decision making. Virtually all commentary on the importance of patient-specific evidence concerns treatment or therapy, presumably because accurate diagnosis is more often viewed as the starting point for treatment rather than as an end in itself. In addition, the longitudinal contact with patients that we need in order to assess progress usually only happens during treatment. Accordingly, this chapter focuses on evidence concerning the effects of treatment with a particular patient.

EVIDENCE FROM CLINICAL PRACTICE

Why do we need evidence from clinical practice, especially if we find compelling (i.e., valid, important) external evidence in support of a treatment decision? Simply because external evidence is obtained with a broader, more telescopic view across one or more groups of patients, so it is usually a much better reflection of the group averages than of the individuals who comprise the groups. Thus, the applicability of the external evidence from even a very strong study to an individual patient will need be tested rather than assumed. As described by Bohart:

> An individual can't be assumed to be a special case of the general—each individual will resemble the general in some ways and will differ in some ways ... the practitioner will always be in the position of what Trierweiler and Stricker (1998) have called the "local scientist," creatively adapting the general to fit with the individual ... [by] adopting an "experimental attitude." (2005, p. 41)

Service providers and clinical settings also have unique characteristics that may prevent a clinical action studied and reported in the research literature from being implemented in exactly the same way by different clinicians in different settings. Thus, according to Wampold, Lichtenberg, and Waehler, "all interventions must be evaluated at the local level as they are administered" (2005, p. 35). In short, when it comes to E^2, clinicians must adapt the features and processes associated with high-quality external evidence to questions about treatment with individual patients.

Honest uncertainty should motivate any effort to obtain strong evidence from clinical practice because valid E^2 requires more than the usual performance monitoring by which competent clinicians show that their patients are improving at the (usually implicitly) expected rate. Such routine progress monitoring generally takes the form of intra-therapy probes (measures of the patient's performance on tasks within the treatment session). When feasible, the clinician may also obtain extra-therapy measures to determine whether skills are generalizing to other domains or contexts (e.g., Fucetola, Tucker, Blank, & Corbetta, 2005). A search for E^2 would occur only if one or more of the relevant parties (patient, clinician, family member, supervisor, third-party payer) expressed honest uncertainty about whether a treatment decision made before or during intervention had been optimal. E^2 is not a synonym for routine measures of patient performance, nor is it reasonable to expect that local evidence about a patient could meet all of the critical appraisal criteria that have been discussed with respect to external evidence. For these reasons, Figure 9.1 is not presented as a critical appraisal form but rather as a checklist of issues to consider in seeking valid, important evidence from clinical practice.

CAPE: CHECKLIST FOR APPRAISING PATIENT/PRACTICE EVIDENCE

Figure 9.1 shows a checklist for appraising patient/practice evidence (CAPE) that summarizes some of the main factors to consider in planning and evaluating evidence about practice with a particular patient. The CAPE form is much less cut and dried than the critical appraisal forms used thus far. It is intended to stimulate planning and thinking about strong evidence from clinical practice, and it should be adapted to fit local conditions (i.e., the patient, treatment, and setting in question).

CAPE: Checklist for Appraising Patient/Practice Evidence

Evaluator: Date:

Foreground question:

    For   (Patient identifier)

    is   (Treatment/condition)

    associated with   (Outcome)

    as compared with   (Contrasting treatment/condition)

Notes on rationale, operational definitions, and so forth:

A. Issues related to the validity of the evidence:

- Observational (A–B) or Experimental (e.g., A-B-A, alternating treatments, multiple baseline)?
- Randomization (e.g., targets to conditions, order of conditions)?
- Stable baseline(s)?
- Adequate length of treatment phase(s)?
- Treatment consistency, fidelity?
- Potential nuisance factor(s)?
- Valid and reliable measures?
- Measures administered with blinding?

B. Issues related to the importance of the evidence:

- Magnitude of treatment effect?
- Evidence of maintenance, generalization, and social validity of treatment effect?
- Substantial cost–benefit advantage?

Validity: Compelling _____   Suggestive _____   Equivocal _____

Importance: Compelling _____   Suggestive _____   Equivocal _____

Clinical bottom line:

Figure 9.1.   A checklist for appraising patient/practice evidence (CAPE).

The Foreground Question

The first step toward obtaining valid and important E^2 is to formulate an FQ that specifies as many of the four PICO components as possible. Accordingly, the CAPE form begins with a space for an FQ, followed by a space for brief notes about the observations or events that led to the question and for operational definitions of the interventions that the clinician wishes to compare.

Imagine that a clinician has provided intervention using the indirect conversational approach she prefers for a child with severe vocabulary deficits. However, after 8 hours of intervention and hundreds of exposures to five high-value vocabulary targets, the child has not been observed to produce any of the new words. Based on her previous experience with the intervention approach and her familiarity with the research literature, the clinician had expected the child to produce all five of the new words spontaneously after this much intervention. The fact that no progress has occurred leads the clinician to uncertainty about the appropriateness of the approach for this patient, and despite her preference for more naturalistic intervention with such children, she decides that she needs to determine whether an alternative approach might be more effective with this child. In particular, she wonders whether the child might benefit more from a more structured, direct instruction approach in which after modeling a word with its object referent the clinician rewards the child for first imitative and then spontaneous naming of the referent.

In this situation, the clinician could simply decide to shift gears to the alternative treatment approach. Doing so would be consistent with recommendations (e.g., Fey, 1988) about how long to continue a treatment without seeing improvement. However, it would probably be hard to judge the relative efficacy of the two approaches in order to decide which one to use—in most clinical situations the better approach for a patient is not a black-and-white decision. Formulating an FQ would allow the clinician to obtain much stronger evidence about the relative effectiveness of the two approaches with her patient.

In this case, the FQ might be worded as follows: *For this patient (P), would a direct instruction approach (I) result in a more rapid rate of vocabulary acquisition (O) than the indirect, conversational approach that has been used for the past month (C)?* In this example, the current approach is treated as the comparison because it is what the new approach will be pitted against. If the clinician had decided to obtain E^2 about two treatment approaches before she had initiated either one in a fully prospective fashion, then she could define either one as the intervention or the comparison.

An FQ guiding an attempt to obtain E^2 about a particular patient could be written to contrast any number of aspects of intervention including different treatment targets, different service delivery models or intensities of treatment, different treatment providers, and so forth. Similarly, a variety of outcomes (e.g., frequency or rate of a target form or target behavior in conditions with varying degrees of support or assistance) could be specified. It is important that the FQ be written as explicitly as possible because being clear about what evidence is needed will make it easier to see how best to obtain it.

Issues Related to the Validity of the Evidence

In planning or evaluating evidence from clinical practice, the intent is to accurately capture information about a particular patient rather than to generalize it to other patients. Accordingly, with E^2, the focus is on internal rather than external validity, and the first section of the CAPE form addresses several influences on internal validity, including study design, measurement quality, blinding, and potential nuisance variables.

As discussed in Chapter 4, questions about an individual patient will require one of several single-subject or N-of-1 designs. Indeed, Janosky argued that when "sound research methodology [is implemented] . . . patient care is a special case of a single subject research design" (2005, p. 549). A great deal has been written about single-subject designs, and this chapter is not intended to replace any of the excellent sources on this topic (e.g. Horner et al., 2005; Mahon, Donner, & Wood, 1996; McReynolds & Kearns, 1983; Sheikh, Smeeth, & Ashcroft, 2002). Briefly stated, all single-subject designs involve measurements obtained over time (or longitudinally) from a single patient or student in an effort to determine whether a clinical or educational action is associated with improved performance or outcome. Backman and Harris (1999) suggested that a single-subject design can be referred to as an N-of-1 trial if efforts are made to increase the degree of experimental control, for example by comparing rate of progress toward a treated goal with rate of progress toward an untreated goal (as in a multiple baseline design). However, the terms are often used interchangeably.

The simplest single-subject design is observational rather than experimental. In it, the patient's performance prior to treatment, known as the baseline, pretreatment, or "A" phase, is simply compared with his or her performance during or after treatment, during a posttreatment or "B" phase. An "A–B" design is similar to the standard approach to monitoring changes in a patient's performance over time during treatment. There is no effort to actively manipulate the treatment that would otherwise have been provided to the patient.

Nonexperimental designs are inherently weaker than experimental ones due to myriad unknown and uncontrolled factors other than treatment itself that could be responsible for any changes in the patient's performance. For example, if an intervention program happened to coincide with a significant reduction in cerebral edema in a patient with traumatic brain injury (TBI), then improved performance might incorrectly be attributed to intervention rather than to improved neurological functioning. Similarly, the frequency of a child's challenging behaviors might decrease because of an unrelated improvement in his or her life, such as the removal of an abusive family member from the home, not the onset of functional communication training. Historical and maturational variables such as these make it impossible to confidently draw inferences about the effects of treatment in nonexperimental studies. For this reason, Horner et al. (2005) argued that the label "single-subject designs" should only be used for studies that are experimental (i.e., involve an active manipulation as defined earlier) and that have additional controls for such threats to internal validity.

Several kinds of single-subject designs involve active manipulations designed to demonstrate experimental control (i.e., a systematic and replicable relationship between changes in the intervention variable and changes in the patient's performance). In a withdrawal or reversal design, the baseline (A) and treatment (B) sequence is followed by an additional baseline (A) phase during which treatment is not provided. Finding that performance increases during treatment but returns to baseline levels when treatment is withdrawn provides additional evidence that the intervention was responsible for changes in performance. The A–B–A sequence can be repeated to further increase confidence in the treatment-improvement relationship.

In an alternating treatment design, the comparison is between two different treatments aimed at the same target. Rather than alternating periods of active treatment with no treatment, following the baseline phase, the two different treatments are administered in alternating order as performance is monitored. This approach enables not only an examination of the individual effects of each treatment but also a comparison of their relative effectiveness. Interpreting results of an alternating treatments study can be difficult when the patient is also experiencing maturational development or physiological recovery, but many clinicians prefer it because it avoids the need for periods without active treatment after the initial baseline phase.

Withdrawal and alternating treatment designs do not provide compelling evidence for interventions that are intended to cause lasting rather than temporary changes. For example, when new vocabulary items or phonemes are acquired during treatment, we do not expect them to be "unacquired" when treatment is withdrawn. Multiple-baseline designs are particularly helpful in such cases. In a multiple-baseline design, two or more unrelated targets of comparable difficulty are measured simultaneously during the baseline phase. Then, intervention is applied to one target while the other (known as a control goal; cf. Fey, 1986) remains in baseline for a specified additional period of time, after which the control goal also enters the intervention phase. Evidence that the first target improves when it is treated and that the control target does not improve until it, too, enters the intervention phase enables increased confidence in a causal relationship between treatment and improvement.

Multiple-baseline studies can also be designed to compare patients with similar disorders who begin the same treatment program at staggered intervals with the expectation that improvements will occur only as each patient leaves the baseline phase and enters the treatment phase. This type of multiple-baseline design across patients rather than across treatment goals might be useful for addressing an FQ about a treatment that is being provided to several similar patients on a caseload or at a facility, although it would require considerable coordination of effort if more than one clinician were involved.

Returning to the CAPE form, any one of these single-subject designs (reversal, alternating treatments, or multiple-baseline) would count as an experimental manipulation beyond a simple A–B or pre-post comparison. Randomization can even be used in the latter two, for instance, by randomly selecting the treatment to be administered first (in an alternating treatment design) or the target to be treated first (in a multiple-baseline design). As usual, randomizing would boost confidence in the validity of inferences about the effects of treatment by reducing the chances that systematic bias or other unknown factors unrelated to treatment could be responsible for the results.

The next question in this section of the CAPE form concerns the need for repeated measurements of performance within the different phases of the single-subject study. Measuring something repeatedly increases confidence that any differences are reliable (i.e., not just due to measurement error). As Kazdin noted, "[W]ith continuous assessment over time conducted before or after treatment, artifacts associated with the assessment procedures become less plausible" (1981, p. 186). There are no absolute rules concerning the number of measurements to be made within each phase, but several suggestions have been made about the length of the baseline phase. McReynolds and Kearns (1983) suggested that baselines could include as few as three measurements, as long as the findings are reasonably consistent across them. However, if performance is variable, additional measurements will be necessary. Only if performance stabilizes will it be possible to interpret any differences between the baseline and the treatment phase. For the same reason, performance during baseline should not be trending in a positive direction at the point when the treatment phase is initiated.

The CAPE also highlights the need to appraise the extent to which the treatment(s) were implemented consistently or faithfully, as well as whether the duration of treatment could reasonably have been expected to result in patient progress.

The next issue with respect to internal validity of evidence from practice concerns potential nuisance variables that might have influenced the patient's performance independent of the treatment administered. Although it might not be possible to do much about them while obtaining evidence from a single patient, remembering to consider factors such as illness, recovery, changes in medication, and other significant changes in the patient's life can help to avoid the potential for false conclusions about the impact of treatment on a patient's performance.

Finally, the quality of the measure(s) that are used to document improvements in the patient's status must be considered in thinking about the validity of patient and practice evidence. Olswang and Bain (1994) provided an excellent overview of measurement issues in clinical practice. First, norm-referenced measures are generally a poor choice for monitoring treatment progress because their broad sweep makes them insensitive to change in specific treatment targets and administering them repeatedly invalidates their norms. Accordingly, criterion-referenced measures of the treatment targets that can be administered repeatedly may need to be developed in order to track change over time. At a minimum, the probe measures should have reasonable face validity, such that a reasonable person would agree that they could provide a true reflection of changes in patient performance over the course of the treatment program.

The next question, about blinding, is a reminder that subjective bias is a significant threat to the validity of conclusions about patient performance, not because any clinician would intentionally deceive but simply because it is so difficult for the person who is delivering the treatment not to see benefits in his or her efforts. Of course, when the evidence comes from clinical practice, the desirability of minimizing subjective bias has to be balanced with the issue of feasibility. Finding, training, and using an independent and blinded observer to measure the patient's performance at various points over the course of treatment requires additional effort and time for both the practitioner and the blinded examiner. One way to make blinded evaluations more feasible would be for colleagues or students to agree to act as blinded examiners for one another as each in turn encounters uncertainty and a need for strong evidence about a clinical decision. But if blinding is not a workable option, even checking to verify that the measurements made by different examiners agree (i.e., showing reasonable inter-rater reliability) can provide a major boost to confidence in the reality of the findings.

Issues Related to the Importance of the Evidence

Because single-subject studies do not meet many of the assumptions required for using inferential statistics (Janosky, 2005), visual inspection has traditionally been the means by which the presence and magnitude of effects in a single-subject study are assessed. When there are enormous and consistent differences between the conditions, the use of this kind of "inter-ocular trauma test" (so called because the differences hit you between the eyes) might suffice. However, the use of visual inspection can always be criticized due to the obvious potential for subjective bias as well as to the mundane fact that differences can be made to look larger or smaller simply by manipulating the scale of the graph on which they are displayed. One way to avoid the problem of bias would be to provide naive raters with graphs of the measures on which the baseline and treatment phases are not labeled and ask them to mark any points that appear to delineate substantially different phases or clusters of data points. If the distinctions between baseline and treatment phases can be identified without foreknowledge, then it seems likely that the differences between them are both real and substantial. Meehl and Yonce (1994) employed a similar tactic to show that naive raters can successfully distinguish between graphs from substantially different distributions of scores. As mentioned in Chapter 5, more objective measures such d_1 and the PND (percentage of nonoverlapping data points) are being explored for use in interpreting results of single-subject studies (Beeson & Robey, 2006; Campbell, 2003).

Evidence that the intra-therapy findings have generalized to outside settings and/or are being maintained after treatment ceases also contributes to judging their impact or importance. In addition, solicited or unsolicited comments by the patient or family members concerning the acceptability or impact of the treatment variations that are being compared contributes to judging importance. Of course, if improvements are noted by people who are naive about either the fact or the type of treatment, then there will be even more credible evidence of treatment effects. The only aspect of importance that cannot typically be addressed in some form in a single-subject study is an estimate of precision in the form of a CI.

The ratio of benefits to harms and other costs for the patient is another aspect of importance that should contribute to the clinical bottom line from a single-subject study. If two treatments are compared but the one with the greatest benefit carries the greatest potential for serious harm, or is so costly as to be inaccessible, then the clinical bottom line concerning the evidence from clinical practice may well come down on the side of the treatment that is less beneficial.

Ratings of Validity and Importance and the Clinical Bottom Line

Similar to the CATE and CADE forms, the CAPE worksheet encourages an overall impression concerning the validity and importance of the evidence from practice with one or more patients that should lead directly to the clinical bottom line, about whether one of the clinical options appears substantially superior to the other.

SUMMARY

As noted at the beginning of this chapter, little guidance is available concerning the use of evidence from clinical practice for E^3BP despite growing awareness of the importance of such evidence for determining whether best current external evidence is relevant to an individual patient in a particular setting. Competent clinicians routinely design and employ systematic, meaningful measures to monitor their patients' progress, and such evidence provides an adequate basis for the vast majority of clinical decisions. However, substantial uncertainty about a treatment decision for a particular patient can and should impel efforts to collect valid, reliable, and important evidence via a single-subject study. It is irrational to expect that many idealized single-subject studies can be conducted in the "hurly burly of real-world clinical care" (Phillips et al., 2001). But when uncertainty about the optimal clinical course for a particular patient is high, even a simple and imperfect single-subject study interpreted with awareness of validity and importance can provide useful evidence for E^3BP.

Clinical decision making seems straightforward if best external evidence and evidence from clinical practice both point in the same direction. What if the two sources of evidence lead to different clinical bottom lines? For example, what if the clinical bottom line derived from best external evidence is that a treatment is ineffective, but there is credible evidence that it is beneficial for the patient? The evidence on the patient's performance should always take precedence in this situation—there are good reasons to doubt that summary evidence from even large numbers of people can be predictive of results for every individual patient. However, regardless of whether E^1 and E^2 converge, there is a third component of E^3BP that must also be considered—the preferences of the patient once he or she is fully informed about the clinical options. Obtaining and using this kind of evidence is the topic of Chapter 10.

10

Appraising Evidence on Patient Preferences

Some people will never learn anything, for this reason, because they understand things too soon.

—Alexander Pope, Miscellanies, p. 346, 1727

The third component of evidence-based practice (E³BP) is evidence concerning the preferences of fully informed patients relating to the clinical options they face. Evidence-based medicine was first defined as the integration of evidence from scientific research and clinical expertise. However, subsequent definitions have emphasized the need to consider the patient's "unique values and circumstances" (Straus, Richardson, Glasziou, & Haynes, 2005, p. 1), and the medical literature contains a growing number of papers that address the need to incorporate this third kind of evidence in E³BP.

As noted earlier, appraising evidence on patient preferences is different from appraising empirical evidence because patient preferences are inherently subjective. This does not mean that we cannot attempt to study private experiences scientifically (Kendler, 2006). But it does suggest that we may need to think even more carefully than usual about how we can create the conditions that will facilitate patients' understanding of their clinical options, including their choice to participate in the decisions about their care. There are two related literatures that can guide us as we begin to tackle the need for valid and important evidence on our patients' preferences.

PATIENT-CENTERED CARE

Kaldjian, Weir, and Duffy (2005) pointed out that the ethical mandate to respect a patient's autonomy can actually be seen as part of the ethical principle of beneficence because it is impossible to act for the good of a patient without understanding what that patient believes will be good for him or her. However, the patient's judgment will be based on a constellation of factors that are not readily accessible to the clinician, including past experience and knowledge (e.g., general life experience; experience with the communication difficulty or disorder; history of prior disorders; outcomes of previous encounters with health professionals; knowledge about the communication difficulty obtained from friends, co-workers, the popular media, Internet-based advocacy groups) and present circumstances (e.g., self-defined goals and needs in the social, vocational, and spiritual spheres; biological, cognitive, social, and financial resources). The impact of such covert and subjective factors on a patient's acceptance, rejection, and compliance with health recommendations has been recognized for years (Borrell-Carrio, Suchman, & Epstein, 2004), and the orientation known as patient-centered care is explicitly intended to solicit and integrate information about the patient's situation, beliefs, and experiences along with the physician's perspective in charting a clinical course.

Patient–Practitioner Communication

Not surprisingly, patient–practitioner communication forms the core of patient-centered care. Patients are invited to collaborate with the clinician in developing a full and complete view of their two perspectives on the patient's situation and needs before coming to a consensus on their respective roles and responsibilities in the therapy process (Epstein, 2000; Stewart et al., 2000). This means that the clinician and client first have to establish a mutual understanding of the nature of the clinical condition and the potential risks and benefits of possible intervention approaches in the broader context of the patient's life. Because patients vary in the extent to which they want to participate in clinical decisions, and because the nature of some conditions means that the available options are few, Heisler, Bouknight, Hayward, Smith, and Kerr (2002) suggested that the level of participation be discussed routinely in the earliest stages of the client–clinician relationship. In addition, initial patients' preferences concerning degree of involvement and other clinical issues also should be monitored periodically because these preferences may change as treatment progresses.

Communication Aids

Communicating with patients about the nature of their conditions and the potential risks and benefits of various interventions is the first step in obtaining evidence on preferences, and the medical literature contains a growing number of studies of physician–patient communication (e.g., Espstein, Alper, & Quill, 2004; Gordon & Daugherty, 2003; Griffiths, Green, & Tsouroufli, 2005). Many authors have noted that it is far from a simple matter to clearly and honestly express the relative benefits, risks, and costs of alternative clinical options to patients even when strong external evidence about them is available (e.g., Cassell, 2005; Mazur & Hickman, 1993; Straus, 2002). Straus described a detailed process that begins by using strong external evidence to calculate an aggregate ratio expressing the likelihood that an intervention will help or harm. The patient's values are incorporated after carefully describing to him or her the benefits and adverse events that could occur following the intervention and asking the patient to rate the positive and negative outcomes in numerical terms. Although the specific procedures described by Straus may not be feasible (yet) for use in communication disorders, the general approach, including asking patients to assign numerical values to risks and benefits, represents a very useful way of approaching the need to communicate such information clearly, systematically, and in terms that patients will really understand.

There is also a growing literature (e.g., Barry, 2002; Deyo, 2001; Ghosh & Ghosh, 2005; Trevana, Davey, Barrat, Butow, & Caldwell, 2006) concerning a variety of health decision aids that can supplement the standard patient–practitioner conference about care options such as audiotapes, videotapes, handouts or booklets, illustrative graphics, cartoons, and computer programs. Rogers, Kennedy, Nelson, and Robinson (2005) described a patient information guidebook regarding self-management for chronic inflammatory bowel disease. Patients contributed to designing the guidebook, which included comments from patients about their experiences with the disease and the advantages and disadvantages of the treatment alternatives, as well as space for the patient to record his or her self-management plan and experiences.

At present, there is not a great deal of strong evidence concerning the impact of varying communication aids on patient care or satisfaction (Epstein, Alper, & Quill, 2004). Because the developers of such decision aids may have different assumptions and knowledge than the patients who will use them, it will be important for the practitioner and patient to discuss the aids in order to verify shared understanding of their contents and implications. Professionals in communication disorders seem uniquely well qualified to develop and evaluate new strategies for communicating in meaningful ways about complex issues such that patients with a variety of comprehension levels can participate in decisions about their care.

There is some empirical evidence concerning the impact of the patient-centered orientation on patients. In the medical literature, Stewart et al. (2000) reported that patients who perceived that they had reached "common ground" with their physician such that the physician understood the patient's unique situation and needs subsequently reported less discomfort and concern as well as fewer diagnostic tests and referrals than patients who did not perceive that common ground had been reached. In psychology, Blatt and Zuroff (2005) found that the quality of therapeutic relationships reported by patients with depression was one of the best predictors of improvement across several measures of clinical outcome. Specifically, patients who perceived that their therapists exhibited empathy ("Wanted to understand how I saw things"), positive regard ("Respected me as a person"), and congruence ("Was real and genuine with me") early in treatment achieved better clinical outcomes than patients who did not have these perceptions. The notion of empathy is particularly relevant here. McMurtry and Bultz emphasized the importance of the clinician's understanding of "what the disease *means* [emphasis added] to the individual in the context of his or her life" (2005, p. 701).

The study of meaning and other subjective experiences presents problems for the methodologies of the quantitative, natural science research tradition. Cannistra noted that one important purpose for intervention is to "make our patients feel better" (2004, p. 1543)—i.e., to improve their perceived quality of life. The qualitative research paradigm offers a number of ideas to use in attempting to acquire strong evidence on patients' experiences and preferences (Slife, Wiggins, & Graham, 2005).

QUALITATIVE RESEARCH

Qualitative research comprises a wide range of methods and approaches, including participant observation, ethnography, phenomenology, and narrative analysis. Brantlinger, Jimenez, Klingner, Pugach, and Richardson defined *qualitative research* as "a systematic approach to understanding qualities, or the essential nature, of a phenomenon within a particular context" (2005, p. 196). Because qualitative researchers often are interested in understanding the meaning of phenomena to the people who experience them, qualitative methods are particularly relevant for obtaining evidence about patient preferences and values.

Overview

There is a vast literature on qualitative research, and many authors have addressed the ostensible conflict between the values of reliability and objectivity, which seem to dominate quantitative research or empiricism, and the emphasis in qualitative research on the valid representation of phenomena that may well be subjective, such as individual experiences, beliefs, and so forth. Some (e.g., Morse, 2005) have pointed out that qualitative research has received short shrift in the evidence-based medicine literature, and this is certainly true with respect to the criteria used to critically appraise external research evidence as well as evidence from clinical practice. However, the themes of validity and importance, as well as replicability and converging evidence, are just as apparent in carefully conducted qualitative studies as they are in carefully conducted quantitative investigations. It is just that quantitative studies concern observable, independently verifiable phenomena, whereas qualitative studies address phenomena that often must be inferred rather than observed directly. As Giacomini suggested, quantitative and qualitative research paradigms "address essentially different questions ... so their findings tend to complement rather than compete as contributions to knowledge" (2001, p. 5; see also Giacomini & Cook, 2000). However, Phipps (2005) noted that professional training programs often deemphasize the training in qualitative research methods that could improve the ability of health care providers to understand their patients' perspectives.

As mentioned before, seeking evidence on nonobservable phenomena puts clinicians in the position of white-box testers whose knowledge and experiences allow them to formulate and test hypotheses about a system they cannot observe directly (e.g., a patient's network of beliefs, assumptions, values, and preferences). Just as with any type of scientific inquiry, we need to use systematic approaches to measuring, analyzing, and interpreting evidence about our patients' experiences and preferences that we can incorporate into clinical decision making.

Methods

How can we acquire and interpret valid evidence about a patient that goes beyond our own beliefs, values, and assumptions? According to Nunkoosing (2005), the interview is the best and most frequently used method for generating qualitative data about the experience of another person. However, obtaining strong evidence about another's experience via an interview demands more than planning a sequence of questions to direct at the patient. The interviewer has to build a relationship that invites rather than demands that the patient provide insight into his or her perspective. As Guyatt and colleagues noted, clinicians require "compassion, sensitive listening skills, and broad perspectives from the humanities and social sciences . . . that allow understanding of patients' illness in the context of their experience, personalities, and cultures" (2000, p. 1293). The notions of common ground and empathy are clearly relevant here, and learning to conduct something more than the perfunctory patient interviews with which most of us are familiar (as both clinicians and patients) is likely to require training, practice, and mentoring.

For patients with communication disorders or differences that complicate the use of interviews, caregivers may be enlisted to assist in soliciting information concerning patient experiences and preferences. Although using a caregiver or patient advocate as the sole source of such evidence is controversial (e.g., McIntyre, Kraemer, Blacher, & Simmerman, 2004), Broer, Doyle, and Giangreco (2005) developed an interview protocol for obtaining the perspectives of students with intellectual disabilities that included clearly defining the role of the caregiver/advocate after first determining whether the student preferred the caregiver to be present during the interview as well as procedures to assure the students of the confidentiality of their responses. Patients with disabilities may need explicit, systematic training to be able to understand their options and to express their preferences. Test et al. (2004) described several studies in which students with a variety of disabilities were provided with training and practice so that they could participate actively in their individualized education program (IEP) meetings.

When evidence from interviews can be obtained, it can be triangulated (e.g., Brantlinger et al., 2005) with other sources of evidence, including careful and reliable observations of patients' behaviors in structured and less structured situations, in an effort to ensure that the patient's preferences are being interpreted correctly. Asking other observers to examine the evidence (after ensuring patient confidentiality, of course) and comparing conclusions is one approach to increasing the credibility of one's judgments. It also may be useful to verify with patients that their statements have been understood as intended, a process known as *debriefing*. A systematic approach to assessing the patient's values, perceptions, and preferences, in sufficient depth and on an ongoing basis, would facilitate the integration of this third type of evidence with external evidence and evidence from practice for E^3BP. However, as Rogers et al. (2005) suggested, it will certainly be necessary to address the organizational and other factors that limit the time available for patient communication. Additional empirical studies concerning the relationship between patient communication, patient satisfaction, and health outcomes (e.g., Heisler et al., 2002; Kaplan, Greenfield, & Ware, 1989) will be helpful in this regard.

CHECKLIST FOR APPRAISING EVIDENCE ON PATIENT PREFERENCES

Figure 10.1 represents a checklist for appraising evidence on patient preferences (CAPP) that might be useful in systematizing communications with patients concerning their understanding of their conditions, their options, and their preferences. This form is not intended to be shared with a patient. Rather, it describes a general process by which evidence of a patient's preferences can be incorporated with external evidence and evidence from clinical practice for E^3BP.

CAPP: Checklist for Appraising Evidence on Patient Preferences

Evaluator: Date:

Foreground question:

For	(This patient, once fully informed of costs, risks, benefits)
is	(One clinical option)
preferred	(Outcome)
as compared with	(Other clinical option[s])

A. Establish common ground through discussions among patient, clinician, and, when appropriate, significant others concerning their perspectives on

1. The nature of the patient's communication deficits
2. The ways in which these affect the patient's ability to achieve participation and other goals
3. The patient's desired level of participation in clinical decision making
4. A plan to monitor these and other issues on a mutually agreeable schedule

B. Prepare information on clinical options, highlighting differences perceptible to the patient:

                                                            Option 1   Option 2

5. What specific procedures, sites, participants, schedules, and so forth are associated with the option?
6. What outcomes (benefits, costs, risks) are associated with the option according to best current external evidence, and what is the quality of that evidence?
7. Is one option substantially superior according to high-quality external evidence?
8. If so, does the external evidence come from patients reasonably similar to this patient?
9. What outcomes (benefits, costs, risks) has the patient seen in previous experiences with the option?

(continued)

Figure 10.1. A checklist for appraising evidence on patient preferences.

Figure 10.1. *(continued)*

	Option 1	Option 2
10. What outcomes has the clinician seen in previous experiences with the option?		
11. Is one option substantially superior according to this internal clinical practice evidence?		
C. Synthesize external and internal evidence		
12. Do external and/or internal evidence strongly favor one of the options, or are both reasonable?		
13. Based on shared understanding of respective benefits, risks, and costs, does the patient strongly prefer one of the options?		
Clinical bottom line:		
Target date for reconsideration:		

The CAPP is structured around a foreground question (FQ) about a patient's preferences among any number of clinical options that could be used to address the patient's needs and objectives. These options could be identified by the clinician, based on his or her knowledge of the professional literature, or they could be options that the patient has learned about through the Internet, the popular press, or other sources. Only two options appear in the sample CAPP form, but columns should be added to match the number of options being considered. Note that the FQ is structured to emphasize that a patient cannot express a meaningful preference among options until and unless he or she is fully informed about the benefits, risks, and costs of the options being considered.

The FQ is followed by a section (A) that is intended to serve as a reminder of the need to establish common ground with the patient by soliciting and discussing the perspectives of the patient, clinician, and significant others concerning the nature and impact of the patient's communication deficits as well as the roles and responsibilities of each party in any course of clinical action. The brevity of the CAPP should not obscure the fact that it may take substantial time and effort to develop a shared understanding of meaning of a patient's communication disorder in the context of his or her life goals, experiences, and so forth. It is important to find time for thoughtful discussions in which there is enough silence for the patient to ponder and articulate his or her perspective prior to beginning to address the specific clinical options that are available.

Section B of the CAPP provides a set of questions intended to lead to an organized description and comparison of each clinical option that faces the patient couched in terms that the patient will understand and care about. It might be useful here to imagine yourself in the role of the patient—what information would you be interested in if someone were asking you to choose among the options? At a minimum, prepare a description of each option's procedures along with logistical information such as treatment intensity (frequency, scheduling, and duration of treatment sessions), location of sessions, and costs of the sessions (both in terms of dollars and time). Supplementing verbal descriptions with communication aids such as pictures, cartoons, video-tapes of mock sessions, or comments from former patients could be very help-ful in this regard.

After describing the options, the next question concerns the benefits, risks, and costs that have been associated with each option according to the best external evidence and the extent to which this evidence is credible. This infor-mation should come directly from critical appraisals of the external evidence concerning each option and the summary ratings of its validity and importance (compelling, suggestive, equivocal). The synthesis of external evidence should result in an answer to the question of whether any of the clinical options is sub-stantially superior to the others or whether (as often is the case) more than one option can reasonably be considered. Furthermore, the question of whether the external evidence has been derived from patients similar to this patient should be addressed explicitly. For example, if the patient suffers from a comorbid condition that was used to exclude participants from research samples, the applicability of the external evidence may be unclear.

The next three questions (numbers 9, 10, and 11) on the CAPP concern any evidence that may be available from clinical practice concerning the various options. First, if the patient has experienced any of the options, it is important to consider his or her impressions of their benefits, costs, and risks, along with those of significant others (such as family members) as appropriate. Second, the clinician's impressions based on his or her previous experience with the options, ideally with this patient but also with similar patients, should be described. Together, the answers to these two questions should lead to a con-clusion about whether the internal evidence from clinical practice strongly favors any of the options.

The last section (C) of the CAPP requests a synthesis of the external and internal evidence in order to determine whether one option is substantially superior to the other(s), as a prelude to the final question about whether the patient strongly prefers one of the options. The clinical bottom line of the CAPP is the place to record the patient's preference among the clinical options at the time when the CAPP was completed. However, because clinical decision making should ideally be a dynamic process that adapts to new information from the research literature, from clinical practice, or from the patient him- or herself, the CAPP form also includes a target date for reconsidering all three kinds of evidence if no new uncertainties or information suggest a need to do so before that date.

ROLE OF EVIDENCE ON PATIENT PREFERENCES

How much weight should a patient's preference carry in clinical decision mak-ing within the E^3BP framework? Wampold, Lichtenberg, and Waehler (2005) suggested that a client's choice among efficacious programs should always be honored unless there is compelling evidence that one approach is substantially superior to the others. At present, the literature on communication disorders contains very few interventions that would meet the standard of substantial superiority based on incontrovertible external evidence that generalizes broadly across patients, clinicians, and settings. Until such evidence is available, the ethical principles of autonomy and beneficence would seem to dictate that clinicians treat high-quality evidence on the preferences of fully informed patients as paramount in clinical decision making, while continually monitoring the external and internal evidence so that the patient is aware of new information that could alter his or her original preference. If clinicians act in accordance with ethical principles and professional integrity and patients are fully informed about the bases for clinical recommendations and the opportunity to collaborate in decisions about their care, there would seem to be little potential for serious conflicts among the three kinds of evidence needed for E^3BP.

11

A Prognosis for E³BP in Communication Disorders

Errors using inadequate data are much less than those using no data at all.

—Charles Babbage, English mathematician

What lies ahead or beyond for evidence-based practice (E³BP) as it has been characterized in this handbook? Predictions are risky, but several trends are emerging that could significantly improve the adequacy of all three kinds of evidence. Some of these trends involve new sources of evidence, some involve better access to evidence, and some involve more sophisticated discourse about evidence.

NEW SOURCES OF EVIDENCE

Two new sources are likely to increase the importance and relevance of the evidence available for clinical decision making in communication disorders. Both involve thinking about evidence on a larger scale than has been common in the past.

Internet-Based Evidence Networks

One criterion for appraising a finding concerns its precision, or the narrowness of the confidence interval (CI) that surrounds it. As discussed earlier in this handbook, the size of the sample from which a finding is derived is an important influence on precision, with measurements derived from large samples generally being more reliable and more precise than measurements derived from small samples. But few individuals have the opportunity, much less the

financial and other necessary support, to mount large-scale studies of important clinical questions by themselves. Even when support is available it may be
impossible to provide compelling evidence concerning a rare clinical condition
at a single site.

One solution to this dilemma, already being explored in medicine, is to
create collaborative Internet-based networks of researchers, clinicians, and
clients around the world who are interested in working together to obtain
strong evidence concerning a foreground question (FQ) of mutual interest. In
the diagnostic arena, for example, Straus, McAlister, Sackett, and Deeks (2000)
reported an international Internet-based study of the diagnostic utility of a
number of putative diagnostic indicators, including interview questions and
elements of the clinical examination, for identifying obstructive airway disease
(OAD). Briefly, pairs of investigators at sites around the world agreed to assess
(independently and with blinding) a series of consecutive patients including
some previously diagnosed with OAD, some suspected of having OAD, and
some who were neither known nor suspected of having OAD. One investigator in each pair administered the gold standard for OAD—spirometry. The
other investigator administered a clinical examination that included items that
were believed to be associated with OAD, such as a history of smoking, self-
reported chronic OAD, wheezing, and laryngeal height. Within a month, more
than 300 participants had been assessed; data were submitted for analysis to a
single site via a secure Internet data entry system. Results showed that the likelihood ratios for individual diagnostic items were at best intermediate, but a
combination of the four most informative elements resulted in a LR+ of 220
and a LR− of 0.13. A replication and extension of this study to a new participant sample has also been reported (Straus, McAlister, Sackett, & Deeks, 2002).
This work provides an intriguing model for efforts to assess and then improve
the accuracy of diagnostic indicators for behavioral disorders generally and
communication disorders in particular. Formalizing multistage and/or multi-
factorial diagnostic protocols and using large collaborative networks to amass
high-quality evidence on the accuracy and precision of each step and each indicator, singly and in combination, should result considerably in a better understanding of the nature of complex disorders and the ways in which they are
and are not distinct from other conditions, a prerequisite for both clinical and
theoretical progress (Dollaghan, 2004b; Meehl, 1997b; Ruscio & Ruscio, 2004).
Similar approaches to obtaining evidence to address FQs on treatment can be
envisioned, although additional challenges posed by the longitudinal nature of
most behavioral treatment protocols will need to be faced before such collaborations become routine in communication disorders. Creating Internet-based
evidence collaborations will require acceptable methods for ensuring that
patients provide informed consent and that their well-being, confidentiality,
and autonomy remain paramount. Methods will need to be developed to minimize the potential for subjective bias to influence participant selection, measurement, and analysis, and approaches to verifying measurement reliability
and procedural fidelity will also be necessary. Finally, authorship may need to
be thought about in a new and more equally distributed way. However, the
Straus et al. (2000, 2002) projects showed that these problems are not insur-

mountable. The potential for conducting such studies in communication disorders is one of the most promising developments on the E³BP horizon.

Practice-Based Evidence Networks

A related development that is being advocated in medicine inverts *evidence-based practice* to call for *practice-based evidence* as well. According to Nutting, Beasley, and Werner (1999), in practice-based evidence, the questions to be answered evolve from the experiences of practitioners in primary care rather than imposed by the theoretical or other concerns of researchers. However, the questions are addressed using methods and controls that increase the scientific credibility of the resulting evidence. Nutting and colleagues (1999) called for practice-based research networks (PBRNs) that reflect the realities of clinical practice and provide a more equitable division of responsibility and credit among investigators and clinicians. They also emphasized the importance of examining not only the predicted but also the unexpected outcomes that occur in the course of a study under naturalistic (as opposed to contrived) circumstances. Glasgow, Davidson, Dobkin, Ockene, and Spring (2006) likewise described practical behavioral trials modeled after the practical clinical trials described by Tunis, Stryer, and Clancy (2003). According to Glasgow and colleagues, practical behavioral trials are designed 1) to encompass a broader range of questions, outcomes, and methods than are randomized clinical trials (RCTs); 2) to enable a more heterogeneous and representative sample of patients and practitioners to be examined; and 3) to address questions about cost and perceived quality of life that have rarely been addressed in RCTs.

Of course, practice-based evidence and practical behavioral trials are not intended to be substitutes for or replace more carefully controlled studies such as RCTs. Rather, they are intended to ensure that there is a clearer link between the questions and findings that arise in the laboratory and those that arise in real-world clinical care (e.g., Green, 2006). More important, practice-based evidence reminds us that the observations and experiences of front-line clinicians (or as Oxman, Chalmers, & Sackett noted, those working "at the coal-face" [2001, p. 1464]) often lead to the most innovative and influential new areas of investigation. Accordingly, it seems that developing an infrastructure and funding sources to support high-quality (i.e., valid and important) practice-based evidence will be an important next step for communication disorders. Initial steps might involve databases of consecutive patient questionnaires (e.g., Pincus, 1997) or short but systematic surveys of independent clinician and parent observations during specified intervals (e.g., Campbell, 1999). Such evidence can be crucial to identifying questions worthy of study in subsequent investigations with better controls. Of course, important questions must be addressed about potential conflicts of interest that can arise when clinicians act as "double agents" (Yanos & Ziedonis, 2006)—simultaneously providing intervention and conducting research (see also Chen & Worrall, 2006). However, avoiding such conflicts of interests is a manageable task, and the benefits of practice-based evidence for the next phases of E³BP in communication disorders seem to be worth the effort.

BETTER ACCESS TO EVIDENCE

Improving the accessibility of external evidence from the scientific literature for speech-language pathologists (SLPs), audiologists, educators, and other behavioral investigators is another crucial development on the horizon for E^3BP. Two developments, one at the level of the individual practitioner and one that will require a profession-wide effort, will be needed to meet this objective.

Individual Actions

Straus et al. (2005) noted that free or low-cost search engines such as GoogleScholar may facilitate access to the research literature, but until the accuracy and comprehensiveness of such search engines are better understood, there will remain a need for individuals to have access to more expensive search engines. University and hospital libraries often purchase institutional site licenses for search engines and databases that can be used by their employees, but individuals may not be aware of these resources or may find that the search engines do not provide adequate coverage of the communication disorders. In either case, it is up to the individual practitioner, investigator, or student to invest time in learning to use the existing resources and in advocating for better or different ones to librarians and administrators. Librarians are an enormously helpful and underutilized resource in the quest for better access to external evidence; many of them are very well informed with respect to evidence sources and evidence quality (e.g., McKibbon, 1999).

Clinicians working in facilities that do not automatically provide them with access to search engines will need to be proactive, vocal, and persistent in their need for ready access to the external literature. E^3BP requires that external evidence be available as soon as it is needed; physicians in many facilities now can use PDAs (personal digital assistants) to gain almost instantaneous access to evidence databases. In such facilities, SLPs and audiologists may need to do nothing more than ask in order to gain similar access privileges. In other settings, however, individual practitioners may need to be prepared to show administrators some of the ways in which improved access can be expected to contribute to the quality of patient care.

Profession-Wide Actions

The National Library of Medicine's Medical Subject Heading (MeSH) vocabulary is a set of more than 20,000 descriptors concerning health sciences conditions arranged in a set of hierarchical trees. Publications entering PubMed are indexed according to their content with one or more of these descriptors, placing them within a hierarchy of related terms so that users can find them without knowing their exact descriptors. The MeSH vocabulary is a very effective system for storing and retrieving knowledge when scientific terms are defined clearly and used consistently. Unfortunately, many terms in communication disorders and related areas are poorly defined, redundant, and/or used inconsistently. Although the MeSH system works reasonably well given this state of affairs, searches for external evidence concerning speech-language pathology and audiology are sometimes complicated to the point of frustration by the lack of a well-specified and consistently applied system of terms and concepts. The need for a profession-wide effort toward a better taxonomy and ontology for evidence on communication disorders is among the pressing issues to be faced in the future of E³BP.

MORE SOPHISTICATED DISCOURSE

As SLPs, audiologists, and other behavioral scientists gain experience in appraising evidence critically, it seems likely that both the quality of the evidence and the quality of debates about its strengths and limitations will continue to rise. However, there are two future developments that will be particularly important in elevating the level of discourse in this regard.

Awareness of Biases

We look forward to a future in which discussions of the nature and value of evidence can be conducted with better awareness of one's own biases and with less stridency. "Evidence wars" in which individuals make impassioned pleas for their own points of view, citing all and only the external evidence that supports them, illustrate exactly the problems that E³BP is intended to ameliorate. As noted in Chapter 1, the complexity of the professions of speech-language pathology and audiology and the difficulty of conducting rigorous studies of many of the questions of paramount importance for clinical decision making mean that reasonable people will be able to disagree about the optimal course of clinical action for the foreseeable future in some if not all of the areas of communication disorders. Such disagreements can be indicators of a healthy and scientifically grounded enterprise in which truth is acknowledged to be an elusive phenomenon and in which the varied perspectives of researchers, clinicians, and clients can be expected to lead to different weightings of the three sources of evidence. Members of each constituency need to engage with open minds and a willingness to give up even their most cherished assumptions and beliefs when strong evidence contradicts them. An appropriate phrase is "positive skepticism"—being committed in a positive sense to one's best understanding of the evidence while being prepared to be shown that stronger evidence supports a different point of view.

Awareness and Availability of Evidence Concerning E³BP

Both critics and advocates have pointed out the need for credible evidence that the evidence-based orientation actually achieves its objective of improved patient care. Increases in the availability of such evidence will also elevate the level of debate concerning E³BP. To date, several studies in medicine show that instruction results in improved performance of evidence-based medicine skills, such as searching for and identifying credible evidence (e.g., Schilling, Wiecha, Polineni, & Khalil, 2006). In addition, Straus, Ball, Balcombe, Sheldon, and McAlister (2005) reported a pre-post study in which the percentage of patients receiving therapies supported by high-quality external evidence increased significantly after attending physicians and medical residents were provided with an evidence-based medicine-training course, materials, and access to electronic evidence-based medicine resources on the ward. However, there remains an enormous need for high-quality evidence concerning the cost–benefit ratio of E^{3}BP, and it is reasonable to expect an increasing number of studies designed to address this question in communication disorders and other areas of behavioral science. The findings of such studies will be crucial to moving the professions beyond current conceptions of E^{3}BP to increasingly sophisticated ones in the future.

SOME FINAL THOUGHTS

I hope that you are feeling excited and confident about your ability to define, obtain, appraise, and apply evidence from external research, clinical practice, and your patients in your efforts to make optimal decisions about clinical care. The intent of this handbook has been to de-mystify the process of thinking critically about all three kinds of evidence and to provide some functional tools for you as you begin to incorporate E^{3}BP in responding to the honest uncertainty that accompanies everyday clinical work.

However, in trying to balance the complexity of some of the information in this handbook with its usefulness, I usually came down on the side of simplicity and ease of use. If you choose to continue your learning about E^{3}BP, you will find more issues, more debate, and more nuanced points of view concerning many of the issues that were introduced in the handbook. For example, not everyone will agree with the decision to expand the construct of evidence to mean something more than external evidence from systematic scientific research. However, a thoughtful discussion about what makes information credible irrespective of its source seems to be imperative if we are to avoid the misconception that E^{3}BP is divorced from, if not antithetical to, actual clinical care. Similarly, there are many additional questions that face us concerning how to proceed when the three kinds of evidence suggest contradictory clinical courses. As noted in Chapter 10, a fully informed patient should have the final say in choosing among clinical options when the benefits, risks, and harms are similar. However, as we begin to accrue stronger evidence that identifies some clinical options as substantially superior to others, we may well face more difficult questions about responding to patient preferences for one of the weaker alternatives. In addition, this handbook has been relatively silent on the issues that surround the integration of evidence on preferences from patients who cannot make an informed decision or from caregivers whose perspectives might reasonably be inferred to conflict with the best interests of the patient. And finally, this handbook has barely touched on the important issue of how we can use evidence not only on the benefits of our interventions but also on their known or potential harms (e.g., Chou & Helfand, 2005).

In short, there is little doubt that the literature on E^{3}BP will evolve and that the ideas in this handbook will need to evolve accordingly. Those who work in the behavioral sciences and have a solid grasp of the principles and processes of E^{3}BP, as well as experience in applying these to actual clinical situations, have a great deal to contribute to its future and to the futures of their respective fields.

References

Almost, D., & Rosenbaum, P. (1998). Effectiveness of speech intervention for phonological disorders: A randomized controlled trial. *Developmental Medicine and Child Neurology, 40,* 319–325.

Altman, D. G., Schulz, K.F., Moher, D., Egger, M., Davidoff, F., Elbourne, D., et al. (2001). The revised CONSORT statement for reporting randomized trials: Explanation and elaboration. *Annals of Internal Medicine, 134,* 663–694.

Amdur, R. (2003). *The institutional review board member handbook.* Sudbury, MA: Jones and Bartlett.

American Speech-Language-Hearing Association. (2003). Code of ethics (revised). *ASHA Supplement, 23,* 13–15.

American Speech-Language-Hearing Association. (2004). *Evidence-based practice in communication disorders: An introduction* [Technical report]. Retrieved December 12, 2004, from http://www.asha.org/members/deskref-journals/deskref/default

American Speech-Language-Hearing Association. (2005a). *Evidence-based practice in communication disorders* [Position statement]. Retrieved April 30, 2005, from http://www.asha.org/members/deskref-journals/deskref/default

American Speech-Language-Hearing Association (2005b). *Background information and standards and implementation for the certificate of clinical competence in speech-language pathology.* Retrieved November 1, 2006, from http://www.asha.org/members/deskref-journals/deskref/default

American Speech-Language-Hearing Association (2006). *2007 audiology standards.* Retrieved November 1, 2006, from http://www.asha.org/about/membership-certification/aud_standards_new.htm

Arnold, L.E., Chuang, S., Davies, M., Abikoff, H.B., Conners, C.K., Elliott, G.R., et al. (2004). Nine months of multicomponent behavioral treatment for ADHD and effectiveness of MTA fading procedures. *Journal of Abnormal Child Psychology, 32,* 39–51.

Atkins, D.C., Bedics, J.D., McGlinchey, J.B., & Beauchaine, T.P. (2005). Assessing clinical significance: Does it matter which method we use? *Journal of Consulting and Clinical Psychology, 73,* 982–989.

Backman, C.L., & Harris, S.R. (1999). Case studies, single-subject research, and N of 1 randomized trials: Comparisons and contrasts. *American Journal of Physical Medicine & Rehabilitation, 78,* 170–176.

Bailey, K.D. (1994). *Typologies and taxonomies: An introduction to classification techniques.* Sage University Paper Series on Quantitative Applications in the Social Sciences, Series No. 07–102. Thousand Oaks, CA: Sage Publications.

Bain, B.A., & Dollaghan, C.A. (1991). The notion of clinically significant change. *Language, Speech, and Hearing Services in Schools, 22,* 264–270.

Barrett-Connor, E. (2002). Hormones and the health of women: Past, present, and future. Keynote address. *Menopause, 9,* 23–31.

Barry, M.J. (2002). Health decision aids to facilitate shared decision making in office practice. *Annals of Internal Medicine, 136,* 127–135.

Battaglia, M., Bucher, H., Egger, M., Grossenbacher, F., Minder, C., & Pewsner, D. (2002). *The Bayes library of diagnostic studies and reviews* (2nd ed.). Retrieved December 9, 2003, from http://www.ispm.unibe.ch/downloads

Baugh, F. (2002). Correcting effect sizes for score reliability: A reminder that measurement and substantive issues are linked inextricably. *Educational and Psychological Measurement, 62,* 254–263.

Beeson, P.M., & Robey, R.R. (2006). Evaluating single-subject treatment research: Lessons learned from the aphasia literature. *Neuropsychological Review, 16,* 161–169.

Begg, C.B., Cho, M.K., Eastwood, S., Horton, R., Moher, D., Olkin, I., et al. (1996). Improving the quality of reporting of randomized controlled trials: The CONSORT statement. *Journal of the American Medical Association, 276,* 637–639.

Berlin, J.A., & Rennie, D. (1999). Measuring the quality of trials: The quality of quality scales [Editorial]. *Journal of the American Medical Association, 282,* 1083–1085.

Berman, S. (2007). The end of an era in otitis research [editorial]. *New England Journal of Medicine, 356,* 300–302.

Black, M.M., & Sonnenschein, S. (1993). Early exposure to otitis media: A preliminary investigation of behavioral outcomes. *Journal of Developmental and Behavioral Pediatrics, 14,* 150–155.

Bland, J.M., & Altman, D.G. (2000). Statistics notes: The odds ratio. *British Medical Journal, 320,* 1468.

Blatt, S.J., & Zuroff, D.C. (2005). Empirical evaluation of the assumptions in identifying evidence based treatments in mental health. *Clinical Psychology Review, 25,* 459–486.

Bohart, A.C. (2005). Evidence-based psychotherapy means evidence-informed, not evidence-driven. *Journal of Contemporary Psychotherapy, 35,* 39–53.

Borrell-Carrio, F., Suchman, A.L., & Epstein, R.M. (2004). The biopsychosocial model 25 years later: Principles, practice, and scientific inquiry. *Annals of Family Medicine, 2,* 576–582.

Bossuyt, P.M., Reitsma, J.B., Bruns, D.E., Gatsonis, C.A., Glasziou, P.P., Irwig, L.M., et al. (2003). The STARD statement for reporting studies of diagnostic accuracy: Explanation and elaboration. *Clinical Chemistry, 49,* 7–18.

Brantlinger, E., Jimenez, R., Klingner, J., Pugach, M., & Richardson, V. (2005). Qualitative studies in special education. *Exceptional Children, 71,* 195–207.

Broer, S.M., Doyle, M.B., & Giangreco, M.F. (2005). Perspectives of students with intellectual disabilities about their experiences with paraprofessional support. *Exceptional Children, 71,* 415–430.

Campbell, J.M. (2003). Efficacy of behavioral interventions for reducing problem behaviors in persons with autism: A quantitative synthesis of single-subject research. *Research in Developmental Disabilities, 24,* 120–138.

Campbell, T.F. (1999). Functional treatment outcomes in young children with motor speech disorders. In A.J. Caruso & E.A. Strand (Eds.), *Clinical management of motor speech disorders in children* (pp. 385–396). New York: Thieme.

Campbell, T.F., & Dollaghan, C.A. (1992). A method for obtaining listener judgments of spontaneously produced language: Social validation through direct magnitude estimation. *Topics in Language Disorders, 12,* 42–55.

Campbell, T.F., Dollaghan, C.A., Janosky, J.E., & Adelson, P.D. (in press). A performance curve for assessing change in percentage consonants correct-revised [Research note]. *Journal of Speech, Language, and Hearing Research.*

Cannistra, S.A. (2004). The ethics of early stopping rules: Who is protecting whom? *Journal of Clinical Oncology, 22,* 1542–1545.

Casby, M.W. (2001). Otitis media and language development: A meta-analysis. *American Journal of Speech-Language Pathology, 10,* 65–80.

Cassell, J. (2005). Miracles of modern medicine/casualties of modern medicine. *Qualitative Health Research, 5,* 555–563.

Centre for Evidence-Based Medicine, Institute of Health Sciences, Oxford. (n.d.). Retrieved October 10, 2001, from http://www.cebm.net/likelihood_ratios.asp

Centre for Evidence-Based Medicine, University Health Network, University of Toronto Libraries. (n.d.). Retrieved October 10, 2001, from http://www.cebm.utoronto.ca

Chen, D.T., & Worrall, B.B. (2006). Practice-based clinical research and ethical decision making–Part I: Deciding whether to incorporate practice-based research into your clinical practice. *Seminars in Neurology, 26,* 131–139.

Chou, R., & Helfand, M. (2005). Challenges in systematic reviews that assess treatment harms. *Annals of Internal Medicine, 142,* 1090–1099.

Cicerone, K.D. (2005). Evidence-based practice and the limits of rational rehabilitation. *Archives of Physical Medicine and Rehabilitation, 86,* 1073–1074.

Cluzeau, F.A., Burgers, J., Brouwers, M., Grol, R., Maekelae, M., Littlejohns, P., et al. (2003). Development and validation of an international appraisal instrument for assessing the quality of clinical practice guidelines: The AGREE project. *Quality and Safety in Health Care, 12,* 18–23.

Cohen, A.M., Stavri, P.Z., & Hersh, W.R. (2004). A categorization and analysis of the criticisms of evidence-based medicine. *International Journal of Medical Informatics, 73,* 35–43.

Cohen, J. (1988). *Statistical power analysis for the behavioral sciences* (2nd ed.). Mahwah, NJ: Lawrence Erlbaum Associates.

Cohen, J. (1990). Things I have learned (so far). *America Psychologist, 45,* 1304–1312.

Concato, J., Shah, N., & Horwitz, R.I. (2000). Randomized, controlled trials, observational studies, and the hierarchy of research designs. *New England Journal of Medicine, 342,* 1887–1892.

Coplan, J., Souders, M.C., Mulberg, A.E., Belchic, J.K., Wray, J., Jawad, A.F., et al. (2003). Children with autism spectrum disorders. II: Parents are unable to distinguish secretin from placebo under double-blind conditions. *Archives of Disease in Childhood, 88,* 737–739.

Davies, H.T.O., Crombie, I.K., & Tavakoli, M. (1998). When can odds ratios mislead? *British Medical Journal, 316,* 989–991.

Day, E., Maddern, L., & Wood, C. (1968). Auscultation of fetal heart rate: An assessment of its error and significance. *British Medical Journal, 4,* 422–424.

Deeks, J.J. (2001). Systematic reviews of evaluations of diagnostic and screening tests. *British Medical Journal, 323,* 157–162.

Demissie, K., White, N., Joseph, L., & Ernst, P. (1998). Bayesian estimation of asthma prevalence, and comparison of exercise and questionnaire diagnostics in the absence of a gold standard. *Annals of Epidemiology, 8,* 201–208.

Devereaux, P.J., Manns, B.J., Ghali, W.A., Quan, H., Lacchetti, C., Montori, V.M., et al. (2001). Physician interpretations and textbook definitions of blinding terminology in randomized controlled trials. *Journal of the American Medical Association, 285,* 2000–2003.

Deyo, R.A. (2001). A key medical decision maker: The patient. *British Medical Journal, 323,* 466–467.

Djulbegovic, B., Loughran, T.P. Jr., Hornung, C.A., Kloecker, G., Efthimiadis, E.N., Hadley, T.J., et al. (1999). The quality of medical evidence in hematology-oncology. *American Journal of Medicine, 106,* 198–205.

Dollaghan, C. (2003). One thing or another? Witches, POEMs, and childhood apraxia of speech. In L.D. Shriberg & T.F. Campbell (Eds.), *Proceedings of the 2002 Childhood Apraxia of Speech Research Symposium* (pp. 231–237). Carlsbad, CA: The Hendrix Foundation.

Dollaghan, C.A. (2004a). Evidence-based practice in communication disorders: What do we know, and when do we know it? *Journal of Communication Disorders, 37,* 391–400.

Dollaghan, C.A. (2004b). Taxometric analyses of specific language impairment in 3- and 4-year-old children. *Journal of Speech, Language, and Hearing Research, 47,* 464–475.

Ebell, M.H. (1998). An introduction to information mastery. Retrieved January 9, 2002, from http://www.poems.msu.edu/InfoMastery

Edward, S.J.L., Stevens, A.J., Braunholtz, D.A., Lilford, R.J., & Swift, T. (2005). The ethics of placebo-controlled trials: A comparison of inert and active placebo controls. *World Journal of Surgery, 29,* 610–614.

Epstein, R.M. (2000). The science of patient-centered care [Commentary]. *The Journal of Family Practice, 49,* 805–807.

Epstein, R.M., Alper, B.S., & Quill, T.E. (2004). Communicating evidence for participatory decision making. *Journal of the American Medical Association, 291,* 2359–2366.

Evidence-Based Medicine Working Group. (1992). Evidence-based medicine: A new approach to teaching the practice of medicine. *Journal of the American Medical Association, 268,* 2420–2425.

Faraone, S.V., & Tsuang, M.T. (1994). Measuring diagnostic accuracy in the absence of a "gold standard." *American Journal of Psychiatry, 151,* 650–657.

Feinstein A.R. (2002). Misguided efforts and future challenges for research on "diagnostic tests." *Journal of Epidemiology and Community Health, 56,* 330–332.

Fey, M.E. (1986). *Language intervention with young children.* San Diego: College Hill Press.

Fey, M.E. (1988). Dismissal criteria for the language-impaired child. In D.E. Yoder & R.D. Kent (Eds.), *Decision making in speech-language pathology* (pp. 50–53). Toronto: B.C. Decker.

Flanagin, A., Fontanarosa, P.B., & DeAngelis, C.D. (2006). Update on *JAMA's* conflict of interest policy. *Journal of the American Medical Association, 296,* 220–221.

Fluharty, N.B. (2000). *Fluharty 2: Preschool Speech and Language Screening Test* (2nd ed.). Minneapolis, MN: AGS Publishing/Pearson Assessments.

Fucetola, R., Tucker, F., Blank, K., & Corbetta, M. (2005). A process for translating evidence-based aphasia treatment into clinical practice. *Aphasiology, 19,* 411–422.

Ghosh, A.K., & Ghosh, K. (2005). Translating evidence-based information into effective risk communication: Current challenges and opportunities. [Review]. *Journal of Laboratory & Clinical Medicine, 145,* 171–180.

Giacomini, M.K. (2001). The rocky road: Qualitative research as evidence. *Evidence Based Medicine, 6,* 4–6. Retrieved September 12, 2006, from http://ebm.bmjjournals.com/cgi/content/full/6/1/4

Giacomini, M.K., & Cook, D.J. (2000). Users' guides to the medical literature XXIII: Qualitative research in health care A. Are the results of the study valid? *Journal of the American Medical Association, 284,* 357–362.

Glas, A.S., Lijmer, J.G., Prins, M.H., Bonsel, G.J., & Bossuyt, P.M.M. (2003). The diagnostic odds ratio: A single indicator of test performance. *Journal of Clinical Epidemiology, 56,* 1129–1135.

Glasgow, R.E., Davidson, K.W., Dobkin, P.L., Ockene, J., & Spring, B. (2006). Practical behavioral trials to advance evidence-based behavioral medicine. *Annals of Behavioral Medicine, 31,* 5–13.

Glasziou, P., Vandenbroucke, J., & Chalmers, I. (2004). Assessing the quality of research. *British Medical Journal, 328,* 39–41.

Glogowska, M., Roulstone, S., Enderby, P., & Peters, T.J. (2000). Randomized controlled trial of community based speech and language therapy in preschool children. *British Medical Journal, 321,* 923–926.

Gordon, E.J., & Daugherty, C.K. (2003). "Hitting you over the head": Oncologists' disclosure of prognosis to advanced cancer patients. *Bioethics, 17,* 142–168.

Green, L.W. (2006). Public health asks of systems science: To advance our evidence-based practice, can you help us get more practice-based evidence? *American Journal of Public Health, 96,* 406–409.

Griffiths, F., Green, E., & Tsouroufli, M. (2005). *The nature of medical evidence and its inherent uncertainty for the clinical consultation: Qualitative study.* Retrieved June 13, 2005, from http://bmj.bmjjournals.com

Grissom, R.J., & Kim, J.J. (2001). Review of assumptions and problems in the appropriate conceptualization of effect size. *Psychological Methods, 6,* 135–146.

Guyatt, G.H., Haynes, R.B., Jaeschke, R.Z., Cook, D.J., Green, L., Naylor, C.D., et al. (2000). Users' guides to the medical literature: XXV. Evidence-based medicine: Principles for applying the users' guides to patient care. *Journal of the American Medical Association, 284,* 1290–1296.

Hamilton, J. (2005). Clinicians' guide to evidence-based practice. *Journal of the American Academy of Child and Adolescent Psychiatry, 44,* 494–498.

Hegelund, A. (2005). Objectivity and subjectivity in the ethnographic method. *Qualitative Health Research, 15,* 647–668.

Heisler, M., Bouknight, R.R., Hayward, R.A., Smith, D.M., & Kerr, E.A. (2002). The relative importance of physician communication, participatory decision making, and patient understanding in diabetes self-management. *Journal of General Internal Medicine, 17,* 243–252.

Henry, J.D., Crawford, J.R., & Phillips, L.H. (2005). A meta-analytic review of verbal fluency deficits in Hungtington's disease. *Neuropsychology, 19,* 243–252.

Herbert, J.D., & Gaudiano, B.A. (2005). Moving from empirically supported treatment lists to practice guidelines in psychotherapy: The role of the placebo concept. *Journal of Clinical Psychology, 61,* 893–908.

Higgins, J.P.T., & Green, S. (Eds). *Cochrane Handbook for Systematic Reviews of Interventions 4.2.6.* Retrieved March 29, 2007, from http://www.cochrane.org/resources/handbook/hbook.htm

Hollenbeck, A.R. (1978). Problems of reliability in observational research. In G.P. Sackett (Ed.), *Observing behavior, Volume II* (pp. 79–98). Baltimore: University Park Press.

Horner, R.H., Carr, E.G., Halle, J., McGee, G., Odom, S., & Wolery, M. (2005). The use of single-subject research to identify evidence-based practice in special education. *Exceptional Children, 71,* 165–179.

Huberty, C.J. (2002). A history of effect size indices. *Educational and Psychological Measurement, 62,* 227–240.

Huberty, C.J., & Lowman, L.L. (2000). Group overlap as a basis for effect size. *Educational and Psychological Measurement, 60,* 543–563.

Institute of Medicine. (1990). *Clinical practice guidelines: Directions for a new program.* Washington, DC: National Academies Press.

Irwig, L., Tosteson, A.N.A., Gatsonis, C., Lau, J., Colditz, G., Chalmers, T.C., & Mosteller, F. (1994). Guidelines for meta-analyses evaluating diagnostic tests. *Annals of Internal Medicine, 120,* 667–676.

Jacobson, N.S., Roberts, L.J., Berns, S.B., & McGlinchey, J.B. (1999). Methods for defining and determining the clinical significance of treatment effects: Description, application and alternatives. *Journal of Consulting and Clinical Psychology, 67,* 300–307.

Janosky, J.E. (2005). Use of the single subject design for practice based primary care research. *Postgraduate Medicine Journal, 81,* 549–551.

Johnson, W.O., Gastwirth, J.L., & Pearson, L.M. (2001). Screening without a "gold standard": The Hui-Walter paradigm revisited. *American Journal of Epidemiology, 153,* 921–924.

Jueni, P., Witschi, A., Bloch, R., & Egger, M. (1999). The hazards of scoring the quality of clinical trials for meta-analysis. *Journal of the American Medical Association, 282,* 1054–1060.

Kaldjian, L.C., Weir, R.F., & Duffy, T.P. (2005). A clinician's approach to clinical ethical reasoning. *Journal of General Internal Medicine, 20,* 306–311.

Kaplan, S.H., Greenfield, S., & Ware, S.E. (1989). Assessing the effects of physician–patient interactions on the outcomes of chronic disease. *Medical Care, 27(Suppl. 3),* S110–127.

Kazdin, A.E. (1981). Drawing valid inferences from case studies. *Journal of Consulting and Clinical Psychology, 49,* 183–192.

Kendler, H.H. (2006). Views from the inside and outside [Letter to the editor]. *American Psychologist, 61,* 259–261.

Kirk, R.E. (1972). Classification of ANOVA designs. In R.E. Kirk (Ed.), *Statistical issues: A reader for the behavioral sciences* (pp. 241–260). Monterey, CA: Brooks/Cole.

Knottnerus, J.A., & van Weel, C. (2002). General introduction: Evaluation of diagnostic procedures. In J.A. Knottnerus, *Evidence base of clinical diagnosis* (pp. 1–18). London: BMJ Publishing Group.

Lancaster, G. (1991). *The effectiveness of parent administered input training for children with phonological disorders.* Unpublished master's thesis, City University, London.

Law, J., Garrett, Z., & Nye, C. (2004). The efficacy of treatment for children with developmental speech and language delay/disorder: A meta-analysis. *Journal of Speech, Language, and Hearing Research, 47,* (4), 924–943.

Lenzenwenger, M.F. (2004). Consideration of the challenges, complications, and pitfalls of taxometric analysis. *Journal of Abnormal Psychology, 113,* 10–23.

Lewis, M. (2003). *Moneyball: The art of winning an unfair game.* New York: W.W. Norton.

Lewis, S., & Clarke, M. (2001). Forest plots: Trying to see the wood and the trees. *British Medical Journal, 322,* 1479–1480.

Lohr, K.N. (2004). Rating the strength of scientific evidence: Relevance for quality improvement programs. *International Journal for Quality in Health Care, 16,* 9–18.

Lonigan, C.J., Fischel, J.E., Whitehurst, G.J., Arnold, D.S., & Valdez-Menchaca, M.C. (1992). The role of otitis media in the development of expressive language disorder. *Developmental Psychology, 28,* 430–440.

Lous, J., Fiellau-Nikolajsen, M., & Jeppesen, A.L. (1988). Secretory otitis media and language development: A six-year follow-up study with case control. *International Journal of Pediatric Otorhinolaryngology, 15,* 185–203.

Mahon, J., Laupacis, A., Donner, A., & Wood, T. (1996). Randomised study of n of 1 trials versus standard practice. *British Medical Journal, 312,* 1069–1074.

Man-Son-Hing, M., Laupacis, A., O'Rourke, K., Molnar, F.J., Mahon, J., Chan, K.B.Y., & Wells, G. (2002). Determination of the clinical importance of study results: A review. *Journal of General Internal Medicine, 17,* 469–476.

Mazur, D.J., & Hickman, D.H. (1993). Patient preferences: Survival versus quality of life considerations. *Journal of General Internal Medicine, 8,* 374–377.

McCauley, R.J. (2001). *Assessment of language disorders in children.* Mahwah, NJ: Lawrence Erlbaum Associates.

McCauley, R.J., & Swisher, L. (1984). Use and misuse of norm-referenced tests in clinical assessment: A hypothetical case. *Journal of Speech and Hearing Disorders, 49,* 338–348.

McGee, S. (2002). Simplifying likelihood ratios. *Journal of General Internal Medicine, 17,* 647–650.

McIntyre, L.L., Kraemer, B.R., Blacher, J., & Simmerman, S. (2004). Quality of life for young adults with severe intellectual disability: Mothers' thoughts and reflections. *Journal of Intellectual & Developmental Disability, 29,* 131–146.

McKibbon, A. (1999). *PDQ evidence-based principles and practice.* Hamilton: B.C. Decker.

McMurtry, R., & Bultz, B.D. (2005). Public policy, human consequences: The gap between biomedicine and psychosocial reality. *Psycho-Oncology, 14,* 697–703.

McQueen, M.J. (2001). Overview of evidence-based medicine: Challenges for evidence-based laboratory medicine. *Clinical Chemistry, 47,* 1536–1546.

McReynolds, L.V., & Kearns, K.P. (1983). *Single-subject designs in communicative disorders.* Baltimore: University Park Press.

Meakins, J.L. (2002). Innovation in surgery: The rules of evidence. *The American Journal of Surgery, 183,* 399–405.

Meehl, P.E. (1992). Factors and taxa, traits and types, differences of degree and differences in kind. *Journal of Personality, 60,* 117–174.

Meehl, P.E. (1997a). Credentialed persons, credentialed knowledge. *Clinical Psychology: Science and Practice, 4,* 91–98.

Meehl, P.E. (1997b). The problem is epistemology, not statistics: Replace significance tests by confidence intervals and quantify accuracy of risky numerical predictions. In L.L. Harlow, S.A. Mulaik, & J.H. Steiger (Eds.), *What if there were no significance tests?* (pp. 393–425). Mahwah, NJ: Lawrence Erlbaum Associates.

Meehl, P.E. (2004). What's in a taxon? *Journal of Abnormal Psychology, 113,* 39–43.

Meehl, P.E., & Yonce, L.J. (1994). Taxometric analysis: I. Detecting taxonicity with two quantitative indicators using means above and below a sliding cut (MAMBAC procedure). *Psychological Reports, 74,* (Monograph Suppl. 1–V74), 1059–1274.

Michaud, G., McGowan, J.L., van der Jagt, R., Wells, G., & Tugwell, P. (1998). Are therapeutic decisions supported by evidence from health care research? *Archives of Internal Medicine, 158,* 1665–1668.

Miller, F.G., Rosenstein, D.L., & DeRenzo, E.G. (1998). Professional integrity in clinical research. *Journal of the American Medical Association, 280,* 1449–1454.

Moher, D., Schulz, K.F., & Altman, D.G. (2001). The CONSORT statement: Revised recommendations for improving the quality of reports of parallel-group randomised trials. *The Lancet, 357,* 1191–1194.

Moons, K.G.M., & Grobbee, D.E. (2002). Diagnostic studies as multivariable, prediction research. *Journal of Epidemiology and Community Health, 56,* 337–338.

Morse, J.M. (2005). Beyond the clinical trial: Expanding criteria for evidence [Editorial]. *Qualitative Health Research, 15,* 3–4.

Munro, J. (1999). *A study of the efficacy of speech and language therapy for particular speech sounds in children.* Unpublished master's thesis, City University, London.

Norris, S.L., & Atkins, D. (2005). Challenges in using nonrandomized studies in systematic reviews of treatment interventions. *Annals of Internal Medicine, 142,* 1112–1119.

Nunkoosing, K. (2005). The problems with interviews. *Qualitative Health Research, 15,* 698–706.

Nutting P.A., Beasley J.W., & Werner J.J. (1999). Practice-based research networks to answer primary care questions. *Journal of the American Medical Association, 281* (8), 686–688.

Odom, S.L., Brantlinger E., Gersten, R., Horner, R.H., Thompson, B., & Harris, K.R. (2005). Research in special education: Scientific methods and evidence-based practices. *Exceptional Children, 71,* 137–148.

Olswang, L.B., & Bain, B. (1994). Data collection: Monitoring children's treatment progress. *American Journal of Speech-Language Pathology, 3,* 55–66.

Oxman, A.D., Chalmers, I., & Sackett, D.L. (2001). A practical guide to informed consent to treatment. *British Medical Journal, 323,* 1464–1466.

Page, J., & Attia, J. (2003). Using Bayes' nomogram to help interpret odds ratios. *Evidence Based Medicine, 8,* 132–134. Retrieved October 30, 2006, from http://www.bmjjournals.com

Pai, M. (2006). Classification of study designs (schematic). Montreal: McGill University. Retrieved January 31, 2007, from http://www.med.mcgill.ca/epidemiology/ebss/Classification_study_designs_version7.pdf

Palmer, C.V., & Grimes, A.M. (2005). Effectiveness of signal processing strategies for the pediatric population: A systematic review of the evidence. *Journal of the American Academy of Audiology, 16,* 505–514.

Paradise, J.L., Dollaghan, C.A., Campbell, T.F., Feldman, H.M., Bernard, B.S., Colborn, D.K., et al. (2003). Otitis media and tympanostomy tube insertion during the first three years of life: Developmental outcomes t the age of four years. *Pediatrics, 112,* 265–277.

Paradise, J.L., Campbell, T.F., Dollaghan, C.A., Feldman, H.M., Bernard, B.S., Colborn, D.K., et al. (2005). Developmental out comes after early or delayed insertion of tympanostomy tubers. *New England Journal of Medicine, 353,* 576–586.

Paradise, J.L., Dollaghan, C.A., Campbell, T.F., Feldman, H.M., Bernard, B.S., Colborn, D.K., et al. (2000). Language, speech sound production, and cognition in three-year-old children in relation to otitis media in their first three years of life. *Pediatrics, 105,* 1119–1130.

Paradise, J.L, Feldman, H.M., Campbell, T.F., Dollaghan, C.A., Rockette, H.E., Pitcairn, D.L., et al. (2007). Tympanostomy tubes and developmental outcomes at 9 to 11 years of age. *New England Journal of Medicine, 356,* 248–261.

Phillips, B., Ball, C., Sackett, D., Badenoch, D., Straus, S., Haynes, B., & Dawes, M. (2001, May). *Oxford Centre for Evidence-based Medicine levels of evidence.* Retrieved September 18, 2001, from http://www.cebm.net/levels_of_evidence.asp

Phipps, S. (2005). Commentary: Contexts and challenges in pediatric psychosocial oncology research: Chasing moving targets and embracing "good news" outcomes. *Journal of Pediatric Psychology, 30,* 41–45.

Pincus, T. (1997). Consecutive patient questionnaire databases: A complementary alternative. *The Journal of NIH Research, 9,* 34, 36, 38–39.

Plante, E., Swisher, L., Kiernan, B., & Restrepo, M.A. (1993). Language matches: Illuminating or confounding? [Research note]. *Journal of Speech and Hearing Research, 36,* 772–776.

Rawstron, J.A., Burley, C.D., & Elder, M. J. (2005). A systematic review of the applicability and efficacy of eye exercises. *Journal of Pediatric Ophthalmology and Strabismus, 42,* 82–88.

Rees, J. (2000). Evidence-based medicine: The epistemology that isn't. *Journal of the American Academy of Dermatology, 43,* 727–729.

Reynolds, G. (2003, March 16). The stuttering doctor's "monster study." The New York Times, p. 36.

Roberts, J.E., Burchinal, M.R., Davis, B.P., Collier, A.M., & Henderson, F.W. (1991). Otitis media in early childhood and later language. *Journal of Speech and Hearing Research, 34,* P 158–1168.

Robey, R.R. (1998). A meta-analysis of clinical outcomes in the treatment of aphasia. *Journal of Speech, Language, and Hearing Research, 41,* 172–187.

Robey, R.R. (2004). Reporting point and interval estimates of effect-size for planned contrasts: Fixed within effect analyses of variance. *Journal of Fluency Disorders, 29,* 307–341.

Robey, R.R., & Dalebout, S.D. (1998). A tutorial on conducting meta-analyses of clinical outcome research. *Journal of Speech, Language, and Hearing Research, 41,* 1227–1241.

Rogers, A., Kennedy, A., Nelson, E., & Robinson, A. (2005). Uncovering the limits of patient-centeredness: Implementing a self-management trial for chronic illness. *Qualitative Health Research, 15,* 224–239.

Rorer, L.G. (1991). Some myths of science in psychology. In D. Cicchetti & W.M. Grove (Eds.), *Thinking clearly about psychology, Vol. 1* (pp. 61–87). Minneapolis: University of Minnesota Press.

Rosnow, R.L., & Rosenthal, R. (2003). Effect sizes for experimenting psychologists. *Canadian Journal of Experimental Psychology, 57,* 221–237.

Ruscio, J., & Ruscio, A.M. (2004). Clarifying boundary issues in psychopathology: The role of taxometrics in a comprehensive program of structural research. *Journal of Abnormal Psychology, 113*(1), 24–38.

Rutledge, D.N. (2005). Resources for assisting nurses to use evidence as a basis for home care nursing practice. *Home Health Care Management & Practice, 17,* 273–280.

Sackett, D.L., Haynes, R.B., Guyatt, G.H., & Tugwell, P. (1991). *Clinical epidemiology: A basic science for clinical medicine.* Boston: Little, Brown.

Sackett, D.L., Rosenberg, W.M.C., Gray, J.A.M., Haynes, R.B., & Richardson, W.S. (1996). Evidence-based medicine: What it is and what it isn't. *British Medical Journal, 312,* 71–72.

Sackett, D.L., Straus, S.E., Richardson, W.S., Rosenberg, W., & Haynes, R.B. (2000). *Evidence-based medicine: How to practice and teach EBM.* Edinburgh, Scotland: Churchill Livingstone.

Sackett, D.L., & Wenner, J.E. (1997). Choosing the best research design for each question. *British Medical Journal, 315,* 1636.

Schilling, K., Wiecha, J., Polineni, D., & Khalil, S. (2006). An interactive web-based curriculum on evidence-based medicine: Design and effectiveness. *Family Medicine, 38,* 126–132.

Scottish Intercollegiate Guidelines Network. (2001). *SIGN 50: A guideline developers' handbook.* Retrieved January 9, 2002, from http://www.sign.ac.uk

Semel, E., Wiig, E.H., & Secord, W.A. (2004). *CELF Preschool 2.* San Antonio, TX: Harcourt.

Shaughnessy, A.F., & Slawson, D.C. (1997). POEMs: Patient-Oriented Evidence That Matters [Letter]. *Annals of Internal Medicine, 126,* 667.

Shaywitz, S.E. (1998). Dyslexia. *The New England Journal of Medicine, 338,* 307–312.

Sheikh, A., Smeeth, L., & Ashcroft R. (2002). Randomised controlled trials in primary care: Scope and application. *British Journal of General Practice, 52,* 746–751.

Shelton, R.L., Johnson, A.F., Ruscello, D.M., & Arndt, W.B. (1978). Assessment of parent-administered listening training for pre-school children with articulation deficits. *Journal of Speech and Hearing Disorders, 46,* 242–254.

Simmerman, S., & Swanson, H.L. (2001). Treatment outcomes for students with learning disabilities: How important are internal and external validity? *Journal of Learning Disabilities, 34,* 221–236.

Slawson, D.C., & Shaughnessy, A.F. (2000). Becoming an information master: Sing POEMS to change practice with confidence. *Journal of Family Practice, 49,* 63–67.

Slife, B.D., Wiggins, B.J., & Graham, J.T. (2005). Avoiding an EST monopoly: Toward a pluralism of philosophies and methods. *Journal of Contemporary Psychotherapy, 35,* 83–97.

Sonuga-Barke, E.J.S. (1998). Categorical models of childhood disorder: A conceptual and empirical analysis. *Journal of Child Psychology and Psychiatry, 39,* 115–133.

Sparks, R.W. (1981). Melodic intonation therapy. In R. Chapey (Ed.), *Language intervention strategies in adult aphasia* pp. 265–282. Baltimore: Williams & Wilkins.

Stewart, M., Brown, J.B., Donner, A., McWhinney, I.R., Oates, J., Weston, W.W., & Jordan, J. (2000). The impact of patient-centered care on outcomes. *The Journal of Family Practice, 49,* 796–804.

Straus, S.E. (2002). Individualizing treatment decisions. *Evaluation & The Health Professions, 25,* 210–224.

Straus, S.E., Ball, C., Balcombe, N., Sheldon, J., & McAlister, F.A. (2005). Teaching evidence-based medicine skills can change practice in a community hospital. *Journal of General Internal Medicine, 20,* 340–343.

Straus, S.E., McAlister, F.A., Sackett, D.L., & Deeks, J.J. (2000). The accuracy of patient history, wheezing, and laryngeal measurements in diagnosing obstructive airway disease. *Journal of the American Medical Association, 283,* 1853–1857.

Straus, S.E., McAlister, F.A., Sackett, D.L., & Deeks, J.J. (2002). Accuracy of history, wheezing, and forced expiratory time in the diagnosis of chronic obstructive pulmonary disease. *Journal of General Internal Medicine, 17,* 684–688.

Straus, S.E., Richardson, W.S., Glasziou, P., & Haynes, R.B. (2005). *Evidence-based medicine* (3rd ed.). Edinburgh, Scotland: Elsevier.

Stroup, D.F., Berlin, J.A., Morton, S.C., Olkin, I., Williamson, G.D., Rennie, D., et al. (2000). Meta-analysis of observational studies in epidemiology. *Journal of the American Medical Association, 283,* 2008–2012.

Sullivan, M. (2003). The new subjective medicine: Taking the patient's point of view on health care and health. *Social Science & Medicine, 56,* 1595–1604.

Tatsioni, A., Zarin, D.A., Aronson, N., Samson, D.J., Flamm, C.R., Schmid, C., & Lau, J. (2005). Challenges in systematic reviews of diagnostic technologies. *Annals of Internal Medicine, 142,* 1048–1055.

Teele, D.W., Klein, J.O., Chase, C., Menyuk, P., Rosner, B.A., & The Greater Boston Otitis Media Study Group. (1990). Otitis media in infancy and intellectual ability, school achievement, speech, and language at age 7 years. *Journal of Infectious Diseases, 162,* 685–694.

Teele, D.C., Klein, J.O., Rosner, B.A., & The Greater Boston Otitis Media Study Group. (1984). Otitis media with effusion during the first three years of life and development of speech and language. *Pediatrics, 74,* 282–287.

Test, D.W., Mason, C., Hughes, C., Konrad, M., Neale, M., & Wood, W.M. (2004). Student involvement in individualized education program meetings. *Exceptional Children, 70,* 391–412.

Thompson, B. (2002). "Statistical," practical," and "clinical": How many kinds of significance do counselors need to consider? *Journal of Counseling and Development, 80,* 64–71.

Thompson, B., Diamond, K.E., McWilliam, R., Snyder, P., & Snyder, S.W. (2005). Evaluating the quality of evidence from correlational research for evidence-based practice. *Exceptional Children, 71,* 181–194.

Tluczek, A., Koscik, R.L., Farrell, P.M., & Rock, M.J. (2005). Psychosocial risk associated with newborn screening for cystic fibrosis: Parents' experience while awaiting the sweat-test appointment. *Pediatrics, 115,* 1692–1703.

Tomblin, J.B., Records, N.L., Buckwalter, P., Zhang, X., Smith, E., & O'Brien, M. (1997). Prevalence of specific language impairment in kindergarten children. *Journal of Speech, Language, and Hearing Research, 40,* 1245–1260.

Tomblin, J.B., Zhang, X., Buckwalter, P., & O'Brien, M. (2003). The stability of primary language disorder: Four years after kindergarten diagnosis. *Journal of Speech, Language, and Hearing Research, 46,* 1283–1296.

Trevena, L.J., Davey, H.M., Barrat, A., Butow, P., & Caldwell, P. (2006) A systematic review on communicating with patients about evidence. *Journal of Evaluation in Clinical Practice, 12,* 13–23.

Truswell, A.S. (2001). Levels and kinds of evidence for public-health nutrition [Commentary]. *The Lancet, 357,* 1061–1062.

Tse, S., Lloyd, C., Penman, M., King, R., & Bassett, H. (2004). Evidence-based practice and rehabilitation: Occupational therapy in Australia and New Zealand experiences. *International Journal of Rehabilitation Research, 27,* 269–274.

Tunis, S.R., Stryer, D.B., & Clancy, C.M. (2003). Practical clinical trials: Increasing the value of clinical research for decision making in clinical and health policy. *Journal of the American Medical Association, 290,* 1624–1632.

Twain, Mark. (1909). *Letters from the earth. Report to the I.I.A.S.* (p. 153; B. DeVoto, Ed.). New York: Harper Collins.

Unis, A.S., Munson, J.A., Rogers, S.J., Goldson, E., Osterling, J., Gabriels, R., et al. (2002). A randomized, double-blind, placebo-controlled trial of porcine versus synthetic secretin for reducing symptoms of autism. *Journal of the American Academy of Child and Adolescent Psychiatry, 41,* 1315–1321.

U.S. Department of Health and Human Services. (2005). Code of Federal Regulations, Title 45 Part 46, Protection of Human Subjects, Subpart A, Section 46.102. Washington, DC: Author. Retrieved October 10, 2005, from http://www.hhs.gov/ohrp/humansubjects/guidance/45cfr46.htm

Vacha-Haase, T., & Thompson, B. (2004). How to estimate and interpret various effect sizes. *Journal of Counseling Psychology, 51,* 473–481.

Valentine, J.C., & Cooper, H. (2003). *Effect size substantive interpretation guidelines: Issues in the interpretation of effect sizes.* Washington, DC: What Works Clearinghouse.

Walter, S.D. (2000). Choice of effect measure for epidemiological data. *Journal of Clinical Epidemiology, 53,* 931–939.

Wampold, B.E., Lichtenberg, J.W., & Waehler, C.A. (2005). A broader perspective: Counseling psychology's emphasis on evidence. *Journal of Contemporary Psychotherapy, 35,* 27–38.

Westwood, M.E., Whiting, P.F., & Kleijnen, J. (2005). How does study quality affect the results of a diagnostic meta-analysis? *BMC Medical Research Methodology, 5,* 20.

Whiting, P., Rutjes, A.W.S., Reitsma, J.B., Bossuyt, P.M.M., & Kleijnen, J. (2003). The development of QUADAS: A tool for the quality assessment of studies of diagnostic accuracy included in systematic reviews. *BMC Medical Research Methodology, 3,* 1–13.

Wilkinson, L., & the Task Force on Statistical Inference of the American Psychological Association Board of Scientific Affairs. (1999). Statistical methods in psychology journals: Guidelines and explanations. *American Psychologist, 54,* 594–604.

Yanos, P.T., & Ziedonis, D.M. (2006). The patient-oriented clinician-researcher: Advantages and challenges of being a double agent. *Psychiatric Services, 57,* 249–253.

Zhang, X., & Tomblin, J.B. (2003). Explaining and controlling regression to the mean in longitudinal research designs. *Journal of Speech, Language, and Hearing Research, 46,* 1340–1351.

Zimmerman, I.L., Steiner, V.G., & Pond, R.E. (2002). *Preschool Language Scale, Fourth Edition (PLS-4).* San Antonio, TX: Harcourt

Appendices

A. CATE: Critical Appraisal of Treatment Evidence

B. CADE: Critical Appraisal of Diagnostic Evidence

C. CASM: Critical Appraisal of Systematic Review or Meta-Analysis

D. CAPE: Checklist for Appraising Patient/Practice Evidence

E. CAPP: Checklist for Appraising Evidence on Patient Preferences

These appendices include photocopiable versions of the CATE, CADE, CASM, CAPE, and CAPP forms. Details concerning the use of each form to guide the appraisal of evidence can be found in the relevant chapters (6–10) of the text, but a brief scoring explanation concerning the CATE, CADE, and CASM forms is included here.

The extent to which evidence meets each appraisal point can be indicated in various ways (see p. 65). One system is described below:

Y (yes)	Evidence meets the criterion in all respects.
Y– (qualified yes)	Evidence meets the criterion in some but not all respects.
N (no)	Evidence does not meet the criterion.
UR (unable to rate)	Information necessary to rate the criterion is not provided; the evidence must be assumed not to meet the criterion.
NA (not applicable)	The criterion is not applicable given the nature of the study.

Based on the appraisal points, overall judgments about (a) the validity and (b) the importance of the evidence should be made using the following descriptors (see p. 77):

Compelling	Unbiased experts would unanimously judge the evidence to be valid or important.
Suggestive	Some appraisal points are open to debate, but unbiased experts would probably agree that the evidence is valid or important.
Equivocal	The evidence can be debated on so many points that unbiased experts might reach opposite conclusions about its validity or importance.

The clinical bottom line indicates whether the validity and importance of the appraised evidence suggests that a change in one's current clinical approach should be considered (see p. 77), according to the following guidelines:

Overall judgment	Validity	Importance	Clinical bottom line
Compelling	Yes	Yes	A change to current practice should be considered seriously.
Suggestive	Yes	Yes	Different clinicians might responsibly
	Yes	No	make different decisions about whether
	No	Yes	to alter current practice.
Equivocal	Yes	Yes	No change to current practice need be considered.

CATE: Critical Appraisal of Treatment Evidence

Evaluator: _____ Date: _____

Evidence source: _____

Foreground question addressed by the evidence:

For _____ (Patient/problem)

is _____ (Treatment/condition)

associated with _____ (Outcome)

as compared with _____ (Contrasting treatment/condition)

Appraisal points

1. Was there a plausible rationale for the study?

2. Was the evidence from an experimental study?

3. Was there a control group or condition?

4. Was randomization used to create the contrasting conditions?

5. Were methods and participants specified prospectively?

6. Were patients representative and/or recognizable at beginning and end?

7. Was treatment described clearly and implemented as intended?

8. Was the measure valid and reliable, in principle and as employed?

9. Was the outcome (at a minimum) evaluated with blinding?

10. What nuisance variable(s) could have seriously distorted the findings?

11. Was the finding statistically significant?

12. If the finding was not statistically significant, was statistical power adequate?

13. Was the finding important (ES, social validity, maintenance)?

14. Was the finding precise?

15. Was there a substantial cost–benefit advantage?

Validity: Compelling ___   Suggestive ___   Equivocal ___

Importance: Compelling ___   Suggestive ___   Equivocal ___

Clinical bottom line: _____

The Handbook for Evidence-Based Practice in Communication Disorders, by Christine A. Dollaghan, Ph.D., CCC-SLP. Copyright © 2007 Paul H. Brookes Publishing Co., Inc.

CADE: Critical Appraisal of Diagnostic Evidence

Evaluator: _____   Date: _____

Evidence source: _____

Foreground question addressed by the evidence:

   For identifying _____ (Patient/problem)

   what is the _____ (Outcome – accuracy)

   of _____ (Index measure)

   as compared with _____ (Reference standard)

Appraisal points

1. Was there a plausible rationale for the study?

2. Was the index measure compared to a reference standard?

3. Was the reference standard valid, reliable, and/or reasonable?

4. Were measures and procedures described clearly?

5. Were measures administered independently?

6. Were measures administered with blinding?

7. Were methods and participants specified prospectively?

8. Were participants recognizable and representative of the actual diagnostic task?

9. Were the reference standard and the index test both administered to all participants?

10. Was LR+ [sensitivity/(1 – specificity)] $\geq$ 10.0?

11. Was LR– [(1 – sensitivity)/specificity] $\leq$ 0.10?

12. Was precision adequate?

13. Was there a substantial cost–benefit advantage?

Validity: Compelling ___   Suggestive ___   Equivocal ___

Importance: Compelling ___   Suggestive ___   Equivocal ___

Clinical bottom line: _____

The Handbook for Evidence-Based Practice in Communication Disorders, by Christine A. Dollaghan, Ph.D., CCC-SLP. Copyright © 2007 Paul H. Brookes Publishing Co., Inc.

CASM: Critical Appraisal of Systematic Review or Meta-Analysis

Evaluator: _____   Date: _____

Evidence source: _____

Foreground question addressed by the systematic review or meta-analysis:

    For _____   (Patient/problem)

    is_____   (Treatment/condition)

    associated with _____   (Outcome)

    as compared with _____   (Contrasting treatment/condition)

Appraisal points

1. Was there a comprehensive and clearly described search for relevant studies?

2. Were clear and adequate criteria used to include and exclude studies from analysis?

3. Were individual studies rated independently?

4. Were individual studies rated with blinding?

5. Was inter-rater agreement adequate?

6. Was an average effect size (treatment) or accuracy metric (diagnosis) presented?

7. Were results weighted by sample size?

8. Was the confidence interval adequately precise?

9. Did a forest plot suggest reasonable homogeneity of findings across individual studies?

10. If not, was a heterogeneity or moderator analysis conducted?

11. Were the results sufficiently relevant to my patient and practice?

Validity: Compelling ___   Suggestive ___   Equivocal ___

Importance: Compelling ___   Suggestive ___   Equivocal ___

Clinical bottom line: _____

CAPE: Checklist for Appraising Patient/Practice Evidence

Evaluator: _____   Date: _____

Foreground question: _____

    For _____   (Patient identifier)

    is _____   (Treatment/condition)

    associated with _____   (Outcome)

    as compared with _____   (Contrasting treatment/condition)

Notes on rationale, operational definitions, and so forth:

A. Issues related to the validity of the evidence:

- Observational (A–B) or Experimental (e.g., A–B–A, alternating treatments, multiple baseline)?

- Randomization (e.g., targets to conditions, order of conditions)?

- Stable baseline(s)?

- Adequate length of treatment phase(s)?

- Treatment consistency, fidelity?

- Potential nuisance factor(s)?

- Valid and reliable measures?

- Measures administered with blinding?

B. Issues related to the importance of the evidence:

- Magnitude of treatment effect?

- Evidence of maintenance, generalization, and social validity of treatment effect?

- Substantial cost–benefit advantage?

Validity: Compelling ___   Suggestive ___   Equivocal ___

Importance: Compelling ___   Suggestive ___   Equivocal ___

Clinical bottom line: _____

CAPP: Checklist for Appraising Evidence on Patient Preferences

Evaluator: _____   Date: _____

Foreground question:

    For _____   (This patient, once fully informed of costs, risks, benefits)

    is _____   (One clinical option)

    preferred   (Outcome)

    as compared with _____   (Other clinical option[s])

A. Establish common ground through discussions among patient, clinician, and, when appropriate, significant others concerning their perspectives on

    1. The nature of the patient's communication deficits

    2. The ways in which these affect the patient's ability to achieve participation and other goals

    3. The patient's desired level of participation in clinical decision making

    4. A plan to monitor these and other issues on a mutually agreeable schedule

B. Prepare information on clinical options, highlighting differences perceptible to the patient:

                                        Option 1   Option 2

    5. What specific procedures, sites, participants, schedules, and so forth are associated with the option?

    6. What outcomes (benefits, costs, risks) are associated with the option according to best current external evidence, and what is the quality of that evidence?

    7. Is one option substantially superior according to high-quality external evidence?

    8. If so, does the external evidence come from patients reasonably similar to this patient?

    9. What outcomes (benefits, costs, risks) has the patient seen in previous experiences with the option?

    10. What outcomes has the clinician seen in previous experiences with the option?

    11. Is one option substantially superior according to this internal clinical practice evidence?

C. Synthesize external and internal evidence

    12. Do external and/or internal evidence strongly favor one of the options, or are both reasonable?

    13. Based on shared understanding of respective benefits, risks, and costs, does the patient strongly prefer one of the options?

Clinical bottom line: _____

Target date for reconsideration: _____

Index

Page numbers followed by "*f*" indicate figures; those followed by "*t*" indicate tables.

Accuracy of diagnosis, 12–13, 81–82
  see also Precision of evidence
Active placebos, 30
Agency for Healthcare Research and
    Quality (AHRQ), 20–21
Alternating treatment
    designs, 118–119
American Speech-Language-Hearing
    Association (ASHA)
  accessing journal articles, 25
  move toward evidence-based
    practice, 1
  registry of clinical
    guidelines, 21–22
Applied research, 63–64, 64*t*
Appraisal of Guidelines for Research
    and Evaluation system, 22
Articles, accessing, 24–25, 134
ASHA, *see* American Speech-
    Language-Hearing
    Association
Attrition of study participants, 45, 71
Autonomy, principle of, 4

Background questions, 10
Base rate of a disorder
  estimating, 86–87
  sensitivity and specificity
    values, 92–93
Basic research, 63–64, 64*t*
Beliefs, *see* Subjective biases
Beneficence, principle of, 4
Benefits, *see* Cost–benefit advantages
Biases, *see* Subjective biases
Blind studies
  clinical practice evidence, 38–39
  diagnostic evidence, 85–86
  internal validity and, 29–30
  single-subject designs, 120
  systematic reviews or meta-
    analyses, 110

treatment evidence, 73
  see also Subjective biases

CADE, *see* Critical Appraisal of
    Diagnostic Evidence
Campbell Collaboration, 19, 20
CAPE, *see* Checklist for Appraising
    Patient/Practice Evidence
CAPP, *see* Checklist for Appraising
    Evidence on Patient
    Preferences
Caregiver interviews, 127
Case reports/case series, 33, 33*t*
  see also Single-subject designs
Case-control studies, 33–34, 33*t*, 36,
    69–70
CASM, *see* Critical Appraisal of
    Systematic Review or
    Meta-Analysis
CAT (Critically Appraised Topic)
    framework, 64
CATE, *see* Critical Appraisal of
    Treatment Evidence
Categorization, in diagnostic
    process, 81–82
Central Limit Theorem, 57
Centre for Evidence-Based
    Medicine, 32
Checklist for Appraising Evidence on
    Patient Preferences (CAPP)
  form, 128*f*–129*f*
  overview, 128–130
Checklist for Appraising
    Patient/Practice Evidence
    (CAPE)
  foreground questions, 116–117
  form, 115, 116*f*
  importance of evidence, 121–122
  validity, 117–120, 121–122
Classification, in diagnostic
    process, 81–82

Clinical practice evidence
  as component of evidence-based
      practice, 2, 114–115
  critical appraisal checklist,
      115–122, 116*f*
  ethical considerations, 41–43
  importance of, appraising, 121–122
  internal validity, 38–43
  microscope metaphor, 114
  practical significance, 61–62
  validity, 38–43, 117–120, 121–122
Clinical practice guidelines (CPGs), 7
Clinical Queries, PubMed, 23–24
Clinical review bias, 85–86
Clinical significance, 61–62
  see also Practical significance
Clinicians
  conflicts of interest, 38, 133
  generalizability of research
      findings to, 45
  see also Subjective biases
Cochrane Collaboration, 19, 20
Cohen's *d* measurement
  calculating, 50–52, 50*t*, 51*t*, 52*t*
  overview, 48, 49–52
  single-subject studies, 56
  systematic reviews or meta-
      analyses, 110
Cohort studies, 33, 33*t*, 69
Collaborative networks
  Internet-based, 131–133
  practice-based, 133
Common ground, establishing with
      patients, 129
Communication, patient–
      practitioner, 124–126
Computer searches, *see* Searches
Confidence intervals
  diagnosis, 99–100, 100*t*
  overviews, 57–58
  systematic reviews or meta-
      analyses, 110
  treatment, 76
Conflicts of interest, 38, 133
  see also Subjective biases
Consent, informed, 42
Consolidated Standards of Reporting
      Trials (CONSORT), 24, 64
Controlled research designs, 33–34,
      33*t*, 36, 69–70
Correlation coefficient, *see* R-squared
      coefficient

Correlational studies, 33
Cost–benefit advantages
  diagnosis, 101
  patient preferences, 130
  single-subject designs, 121
  treatment, 76–77
Criterion-referenced tests
  single-subject designs, 120
  validity of, 31, 39–40, 73
Critical Appraisal of Diagnostic
      Evidence (CADE)
  appraisal points, 84–87, 99–101
  compared to Critical Appraisal of
      Treatment Evidence, 82
  example study, 101–103, 102*t*, 103*f*
  foreground questions, 83–84
  form, 64–66, 83–84, 84*f*, 103*f*
  likelihood ratios, 87, 92–95, 94*t*,
      96*f*, 97–99
  nomograms, 95, 96*f*, 97
  sensitivity and specificity, 87,
      91–92, 99*t*
  2x2 tables, 88–91, 88*t*, 89*t*, 90*t*, 91*t*
  validity and importance, 101
Critical Appraisal of Systematic
      Review or Meta-Analysis
      (CASM)
  appraisal points, 107–112
  form, 64–66, 106–107, 106*f*
Critical Appraisal of Treatment
      Evidence (CATE)
  appraisal points, 68–77
  example studies, 68*t*, 78–80, 78*t*,
      79*f*
  form, 64–66, 67*f*, 79*f*
  validity and importance, 72–73,
      75, 77
Cross-sectional studies, 33, 33*t*
Current best evidence, *see* External
      evidence

D value, *see* Cohen's *d* measurement
Debriefing, 127
Decision making
  evidence-based practice and, 7–8
  patient preferences, 130–131
  patient-centered care, 124–126
  uncertainty, 3, 8
  see also Questions, formulating
Diagnostic process
  accuracy of, 12–13, 81–82

as classification, 13, 81–82
critical appraisal of evidence, 83–87, 83*f*, 99–101
foreground questions, 12–13, 83–84
likelihood ratios, 87, 92–95, 94*t*, 96*f*, 97–99
nomograms, 95, 96*f*, 97
sensitivity and specificity, 87, 91–92, 99*t*
2x2 tables, 88–91, 88*t*, 89*t*, 90*t*, 91*t*
validity and importance, 101
Differential diagnosis
classification concept, 81–82
2x2 tables, 90–91, 91*t*
see also Diagnostic process
Differential verification bias, 87
Double-blind studies, 29–30

EBM Toolbox, 99–100
Effect size (ES)
Cohen's *d*, 49–52, 50*t*, 51*t*, 52*t*, 56
odds ratio, 54–55, 55*t*
overview, 47–49
R-squared coefficient, 53–54
single-subject designs, 55–56
systematic reviews and meta-analyses, 110
treatment evidence, 75
Effectiveness, of treatment, 60
Efficacy, of treatment, 60
Electronic searches, *see* Searches
Empathy, 125, 127
ES, *see* Effect size
Ethical principles, 4, 41–43
Evidence-based medicine
definition, 2
instruction in, 135–136
Evidence-based practice (E³BP)
clinical decision making and, 7–8
components of, 2–3
criticisms of, 1–2
need for evidence, 135–136
preconditions to, 3–4
trends, 131–136
Evidence-rating schemes, 5–7, 6*t*
Experimental research designs
internal validity and, 32, 33–34, 36
single-subject studies, 118–120
treatment studies, 69–70
types of, 33*t*

External evidence
applied versus basic research, 63–64, 64*t*
effect size, 47–56, 50*t*, 51*t*, 52*t*, 55*t*
external validity, 43–45
formulating foreground questions about, 9–13
internal validity, 28–38
practical significance, 60–61
precision, 57–59
PubMed searches, 5, 19, 23–26
shortcuts to finding, 17–19, 18*t*
telescope metaphor, 113–114
see also Importance of evidence; Validity
External validity, 28, 43–45

Face validity, 39, 73
Foreground questions (FQs)
about external evidence, 9–13
clinical practice evidence, 13–14, 116–117
diagnostic evidence, 12–13, 83–84
patient preferences, 14–15, 128–129
systematic review or meta-analysis, 107
treatment evidence, 66–67
Forest (Forrest) plots, 58–59, 59*f*
"4S" search hierarchy, 19
FQs, *see* Foreground questions
Full-text articles, accessing, 24–25
Functional outcomes, 61
Funnel plots, 108, 108*f*

Generalizability, *see* External validity
Gold standards, 83–86
GoogleScholar, 134
Guidelines
clinical practice guidelines (CPGs), 7
online sources, 20–22

Harms, *see* Cost–benefit advantages
Heterogeneity analysis, 110–112
Homogeneity analysis, 110–112
Human subjects, ethical conduct and, 41–43

Importance of evidence
  clinical practice, 121–122
  diagnosis, 101
  effect size and, 47–56
  practical significance, 60–62
  precision and, 56–60
  single-subject designs, 121–122
  systematic reviews and meta-
      analyses, 112
  treatment, 75, 77
Index standards, comparing to
      reference standards, 83–86
Individual investigators, as source of
      external evidence, 22
Informed consent, 42
Institute of Education Sciences What
      Works Clearinghouse, 22
Institutional Review Board (IRB), 42
Intention-to-treat principle, 71
Internal evidence, see Clinical
      practice evidence
Internal validity
  clinical practice evidence, 38–43,
      117–120
  external evidence, 28–38
  nuisance variables, 36–37, 43
  overview, 28
  research design and, 31–36, 40–43
  statistical significance and, 37–38
  subjective bias and, 28–30, 38–39
International Classification of
      Functioning, Disability and
      Health of the World Health
      Organization, 61
Internet searches
  PubMed, 5, 19, 23–26
  search engines, 134
  shortcuts, 17–19, 18t
  strategies and sequences, 19–23
Internet-based evidence networks,
      131–133
Intervention, see Treatment
Interviews, patient, 127–128
IRB, see Institutional Review Board

Journal articles, accessing, 24–25, 134
Justice, principle of, 4

Levels of evidence, 5–6, 6t
Libraries, 134

Likelihood ratios, 87, 92–95, 94t, 96f,
      97–99
Literature, accessing, 24–25, 134
Longitudinal designs, see Single-
      subject designs

Malleus Malleficarum, 4
Masking, see Blind studies
Matched groups research designs, 36
MCID, see Minimal clinically
      important difference
Measurement error, 39–40
Measurement, quality of, see Quality
      of evidence
Medical College of Georgia,
      definition of formal
      research, 41
Medical Subject Headings
      (MeSH), 23, 134–135
Meta-analyses
  compared to systematic
      reviews, 105
  critical appraisal of, 106–112, 106f
  forest plots, 58, 59f, 110–112, 111f
  funnel plots, 108, 108f
  purposes of, 7, 22
Minimal clinically important
      difference (MCID), 60
Moderator analysis, 110–112
Multiple baseline designs, 33t, 40–41,
      119
My NCBI, 24
National Center for Biotechnology
      Information (NCBI),
      PubMed, 5, 19, 23–26
National Guideline
      Clearinghouse, 20–21
National Library of Medicine
      Medical Subject Headings
      (MeSH), 23, 134–135
  PubMed, 5, 19, 23–26
NCBI, see National Center for
      Biotechnology Information
Networks
  Internet-based, 131–133
  practice-based, 133
N-of-1 trials, see Single-subject
      designs
Nomograms, 95, 96f, 97
Nonexperimental research designs
  external validity, 43–44

internal validity, 32, 33, 34–35
  single-subject studies, 118
Nonmaleficence, principle of, 4
Norm-referenced tests
  single-subject designs, 120
  validity of, 30–31, 39, 72
Nuisance variables
  internal validity and, 36–37, 43
  practice evidence, 43
  single-subject designs, 120
  treatment evidence, 74

Objectivity, *see* Subjective biases
Observational research designs, *see*
  Nonexperimental research
  designs
Observer drift, 38
Odds ratios
  overview, 48, 54–55, 55*t*
  systematic reviews and meta-
    analyses, 110
On-line searches, *see* Searches
Opinions, *see* Subjective biases
Outcomes
  in foreground questions, 10
  functional, 61
Oxford Centre for Evidence-Based
  Medicine
  glossary, 32
  levels of evidence, 5–6, 6*t*

Parallel groups, 69
Patient interviews, 127–128
Patient preferences
  as component of evidence-based
    practice, 2–3, 123, 130–131
  critical appraisal checklist,
    128–130, 128*f*–129*f*
  patient-centered care, 123–126
  qualitative research, 126–128
  white box metaphor, 114
Patient/practice evidence, *see*
  Clinical practice evidence
Patients
  ethical considerations, 41–43
  patient-centered care, 123–126
  protection of, 4
Patient-specific evidence, *see* Clinical
  practice evidence

PBRNs, *see* Practice-based research
  networks
Pearson's r, *see* R-squared
  coefficient
Percentage of nonoverlapping data
  points (PND), 121
PICO, *see* Foreground questions
Placebos, 30
Positive skepticism, 135
Practical significance
  of clinical practice evidence,
    61–62
  of external evidence, 60–61
Practice evidence, *see* Clinical
  practice evidence
Practice-based research networks
  (PBRNs), 133
Precision of evidence
  confidence intervals, 57–58
  diagnostic evidence, 99–100,
    100*t*
  forest (Forrest) plots, 58–59, 59*f*
  systematic reviews and meta-
    analyses, 110
  treatment evidence, 75–76, 76*t*
Predictive values, 87
Pre-post study designs, 40
Presentations, as source of external
  evidence, 18
Prevalence studies, 33
Probability
  pretest and posttest, 95, 96*f*, 97
  see also Effect size; Likelihood
    ratios; Precision
Probe measures, *see* Criterion-
  referenced tests
Proportions tests, 110
Prospective studies
  diagnosis, 86
  internal validity and, 35, 36
  treatment, 70
PubMed, 5, 19, 23–26

Qualitative research, 126–128
Quality of evidence
  clinical practice evidence, 39–40
  evidence-rating schemes, 5–7, 6*t*
  external evidence, 30–31
  single-subject designs, 120
  see also Importance of evidence;
    Validity

Questions, formulating
    about external evidence, 9–13
    see also Foreground questions

Randomized research designs, 36
    external validity, 44–45
    internal validity, 31–32
    single-subject studies, 41
    treatment studies, 70
Rating schemes for external
        evidence, 5–7, 6*t*
Receiver operating curves, 87, 110
Reference standards, comparing to
        index standards, 83–86
Reliability
    criterion-referenced tests, 39–40, 73
    standardized tests, 31
    treatment evidence, 72–73
Remediation, *see* Treatment
Repeated measurements, 119–120
Research articles, accessing,
        24–25, 134
Research design
    applied versus basic, 63–64, 64*t*
    clinical practice evidence
            and, 40–43
    ethical conduct, 41–43
    external evidence and, 31–36
    external validity, 43–45
    internal validity, 31–36, 40–43
    rating external evidence, 6
    treatment studies, 69–70
Retrospective studies, 35, 70
Reversal research designs, 118
Review groups, as source of external
        evidence, 19–22
Risks, *see* Cost–benefit advantages
R-squared coefficient
    overview, 48, 53–54
    systematic reviews or meta-
            analyses, 110

Sample size, 76, 76t
Scottish Intercollegiate Guidelines
        Network (SIGN), 64
Screening
    classification concept, 81–82
    formulating foreground
            questions, 12–13

reference standards, 90
    see also Diagnostic process
Searches
    PubMed, 5, 19, 23–26
    search engines, 134
    shortcuts, 17–19, 18*t*
    strategies and sequences, 19–23
Sensitivity, 87, 91–92, 99*t*
SIGN, *see* Scottish Intercollegiate
        Guidelines Network
Significance, statistical, 37–38, 47
    see also Confidence intervals;
            Effect size
Single-blind studies, 29–30
Single-subject designs
    effect size, 55–56
    influence on evidence-based
            practice, 2
    validity, 40–41, 117–120
Specificity, 87, 91–92, 99*t*
Spectrum bias, 86–87
Standard deviations, 49–50
Standard errors, 57–58
Standardized tests, *see* Norm-
        referenced tests
STARD, 24
Statistical power, 38, 74–75
    see also Effect size; Precision
Statistical significance, 37–38, 47
    see also Confidence intervals;
            Effect size
Study design, *see* Research design
Subjective biases
    awareness of, 3–4
    clinical review bias, 85–86
    differential verification bias, 87
    disagreements among
            professionals, 135
    in external evidence, 18–19
    internal validity and, 28–30, 38–39
    single-subject designs, 120, 121
    spectrum bias, 86–87
    see also Blind studies
Substantive significance, *see*
        Importance of evidence
Surveillance studies, 33
Systematic reviews
    compared to meta-analyses, 105
    critical appraisal of, 106–112, 106*f*
    funnel plots, 108, 108*f*
    purposes of, 7, 22

Textbooks, as source of external
     evidence, 18–19
Therapy, *see* Treatment
Treatment
     critical appraisal of, 66–77, 66*f*
     efficacy versus effectiveness, 60
     example studies, 68*t*, 78–80, 78*t*,
          79*f*
     fidelity, 45, 72
     validity and importance, 72–73, 75,
          77
Triple-blind studies, 29–30
2x2 tables for diagnostic evidence,
     88–91, 88*t*, 89*t*, 90*t*, 91*t*
Type I errors, 38
Type II errors, 38

Uncertainty
     in clinical decision making, 3, 8
     as motivation for obtaining clinical
          practice evidence, 115, 122
Uncontrolled studies, 33, 33*t*
     see also Nonexperimental research
          designs
University of Iowa, "Monster Study"
     of stuttering, 42–43
U.S. Department of Education, What
     Works Clearinghouse, 22
U.S. Department of Health and
     Human Services

Agency for Healthcare Research
     and Quality, 20–21
definition of research, 41
U.S. National Center for
     Biotechnology Information
     (NCBI), PubMed, 5, 19, 23–26

Validity
     clinical practice evidence, 38–43,
          117–120, 121–122
     concept of, 27–28
     diagnostic evidence, 101
     external, 43–45
     external evidence, 28–38
     internal, 28–43
     single-subject designs, 121–122
     systematic reviews and meta-
          analyses, 112
     treatment evidence, 72–73, 77
Variables, nuisance, 36–37, 43, 74
Verification bias, 87
What Works Clearinghouse, 22
Withdrawal research designs, 118
Workshops, as source of external
     evidence, 18
World Health Organization,
     International Classification of
     Functioning, Disability and
     Health, 61